Gastroparesis

By

Lynne D M Noble M.Ed., BSc (Hons)

Dip. Nutritional Medicine,

Diploma Mental Health Care

Independently published 2019

Note: parts of this book are reproduced in 'Alleviating Symptoms of EDS.'

Contents

About the Author

Lynne Noble was born in 1953 in Huddersfield, West Yorkshire. From a very early age, Lynne showed an interest in nutrition and genetics avidly reading any books that she could get her hands on at the time.

Initially, Lynne studied orthopaedics but events led her to work with the elderly mentally infirm. Here, her interest in neurodegenerative disorders and pain syndromes developed.

Lynne undertook rigorous programmes of study, completing her Cert Ed., (FE) BSc (Hons) and Adv. Dip Education simultaneously before moving onto her M.Ed.

From there she took further demanding programmes in Human Nutrition, Pharmacology, Neuroscience, Genetics and Immunology. During this time, she was given many prestigious awards for her academic work. It was noted then that Lynne was not afraid of tackling difficult subjects.

She began her law degree but ill health prevented her from pursuing this. However, in this time, she moved from being a foster parent to adoptive parent.

She has been instrumental in setting up projects in the community for disadvantaged groups.

She is a member of the Guild of Health Writers.

Now retired, she lives in a picturesque village in West Yorkshire with her husband. She enjoys gardening, watching her husband bowling and researching.

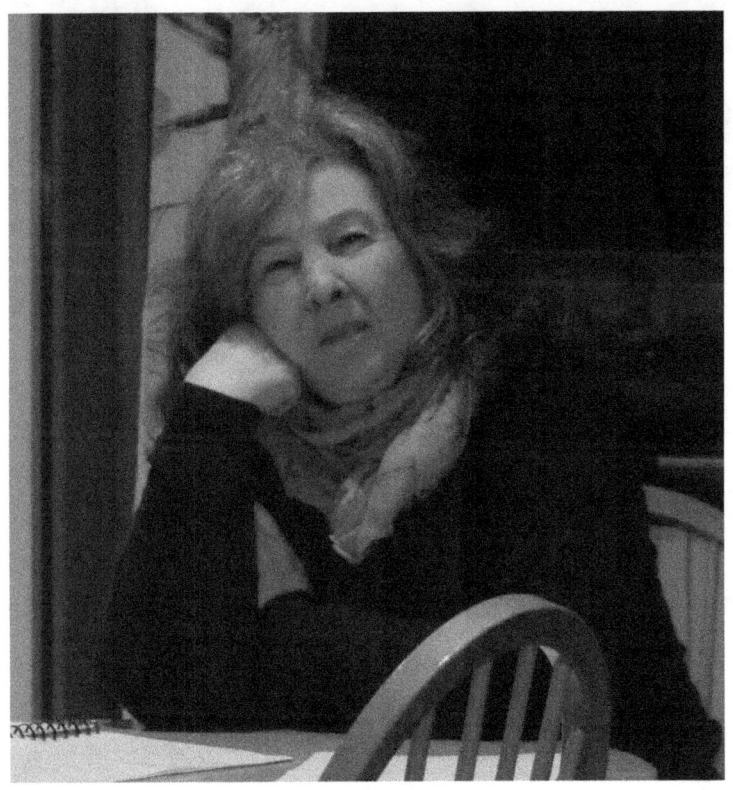

Author Lynne Noble at home

https://quintessentiallylynne.weebly.com/nutritional-medicine.html

Preface

I have received a lot of posts recently that have been sent to my social media sites, reminding me that this month is gastroparesis awareness month. Gastroparesis is one of the myriad of debilitating symptoms that no one appears to have heard of unless, of course, you have a condition like Elhers Danlos Syndrome (EDS), multiple sclerosis or another neurodegenerative disorder like Alzheimer's disease. Then it is quite likely that not only will you have heard of it but that you are likely to be experiencing the effects of it.

In fact, people with chronic conditions tend to be experts on their conditions and often inform those medics who are looking after their health about treatment and prescription medications.

Even so, gastroparesis is still seen as a distressing and debilitating condition that seems to be difficult to manage. It is referred to as a subclinical disorder. It does not have recognisable clinical findings- that is, it does not have identifiable signs and symptoms that can be pinned down to a specific deficiency in the mechanisms of the digestive system. At best, the lack of a mechanical obstruction may lead a medic to explore the possibility of gastroparesis.

While nutritional factors play a huge part in alleviating symptoms of gastroparesis, this does not happen overnight. Further, a little detective work needs to be undertaken. There are many nutrients and medications that can cause gastroparesis, too. Some will probably surprise you as they are not generally raised by medics when they are prescribing medication.

It is not unknown that for every drug prescribed it requires a further two to deal with the side effects. Therefore, this book does not recommend over the counter or prescription drugs. This book helps you examine some common causes of gastroparesis that you may not have known about. Following on from this, nutritional substances – and more importantly, why they work – are introduced.

It is the dietary changes that will have the greatest impact on this condition.

As always, I do not propose increasing prescribed medication to cope with symptoms. Bespoke nutrition is regenerating, not degenerating so there should be less need for medication as time goes on. Besides, prescribed medication has so many side effects that much of the patient's medication is prescribed to reduce the side effects of the medication given in the first place. It is prescribed to mask symptoms and does not deal with the underlying cause.

What I prescribe is an understanding of the processes underpinning a disease and recommend bespoke nutrition to address it. Some of the beneficial effects will be felt almost immediately and others will take time to manifest themselves but they **will** manifest themselves if the diet is adhered to.

I am aware that a low fibre diet is recommended for those with gastroparesis and I understand the reasons why this is recommended. A low fibre diet appears far gentler but in some respects can make matters worse. The gut is meant to 'grip' on fibre. It helps peristalsis. Constipation and gastroparesis tend to be associated

In the end, every individual has to decide what works best for them. However, it may be that when you change some areas that are contributing to your gastroparesis the need for a low fibre diet dissipates slowly. Some dietary fibre is required for a healthy gut biome. A poor gut microbiome will result in bacterial overgrowth and this, in itself can cause gastroparesis.

Although gastroparesis is difficult to live with and difficult to treat, it can be done but the causes underpinning this condition need to be investigated. Each individual that has gastroparesis may have one – or a number – of causes contributing to their condition. This is why there cannot be a 'one size fits all' response to any condition. The human body is more complex than that.

I believe that it always helps to have a simple understanding of the part of the body that appears to be malfunctioning so, with that in mind, I have included some simple information.

I have included other digestive conditions - where peristaltic activity is reduced – that may impact on gastroparesis. The interconnectedness of the digestive system is not in doubt and it would be foolish to look at gastroparesis in isolation from the rest of the digestive system.

The Stomach and its hormonal influences

The stomach has three main digestive functions. These are:

- The storage of food
- The breakdown of food (chyme) achieved by enzymes or during the mechanical grinding of food by the stomach muscles.
- The slow release of the chyme to the duodenum. The speed of the release very much depends on the small intestine's ability to digest and absorb the chyme.

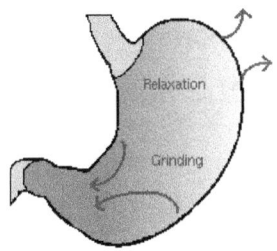

The upper part of the stomach is known as the proximal stomach. It is characterised by weak contractions and storage of food. The muscle is quite thin compared to the distal stomach.

The distal stomach consists of the antrum and pylorus muscle. The muscular wall is thick and powerful. This area of the stomach is concerned with the digestion of food through the action of enzymes that help break food down. The thick muscular walls grind the food and break it down that way.

This lower area of the stomach also regulates the rate at which the partially digested food (known as chyme) is allowed through into the duodenum.

The Migrating Myoelectric Complex (MMC) better known as the Housekeeper.

After food has been digested and absorbed, contractions still continue in the empty stomach and small intestine. These are managed by the MMC also known as the Housekeeper.

These contractions move down the full length of the gastrointestinal tract taking about two hours to complete this process. On completion of this clearing out process, another wave of contractions begins.

Peristalsis

• series of involuntary wave-like muscle contractions which move food along the digestive tract

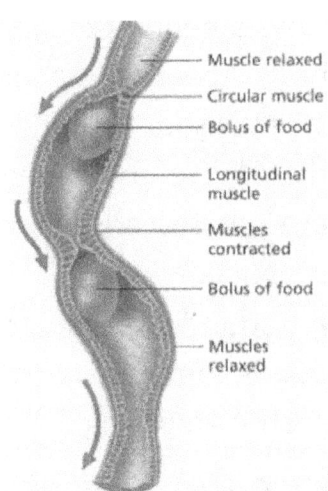

Muscle relaxed

Circular muscle

Bolus of food

Longitudinal muscle

Muscles contracted

Bolus of food

Muscles relaxed

1

Now we can already begin to see that a number of things can go wrong with this process. For example,

- The muscular function in the distal part of the stomach needs to be working properly. The food needs to have been

---

[1] https://healthjade.net/peristalsis/

broken down enough to pass through the pylorus muscle.

- The pylorus muscle must be in a ready state to allow the above.
- Cholinergic stimuli govern the Housekeeper function. Therefore, there has to be enough acetylcholine synthesised to initiate the contractions that move food along. Many diseases are characterised by a deficiency of acetylcholine.
- Intraduodenal fat (that is, fat in the duodenum) is a potent inhibitor of gastric emptying

However, this is far too simplistic a picture of the workings of the digestive system. There are a number of hormonal influences that regulate the process – some by inhibiting gut motility and some by increasing it.

Here's some of the more common ones you are likely to come across:

Table showing gastric hormones and their mode of action

Gastric hormone	Function
cholecystokinin	It facilitates digestion in the small intestine by delivering enzymes from the pancreas and gall bladder. It relaxes the proximal stomach and contracts the pyloric sphincter. Both of these actions inhibit gastric emptying
Secretin	Secretin is released in response to acid in the small intestine. It stimulates the pancreas and bile ducts to release bicarbonate. This neutralises acid and inhibits intestinal motility.
Gastrin	Works in a similar

	way to cholecystokinin. Thus it helps relax the upper part of the stomach and enhance contraction in the distal stomach
Motilin	Promotes gastric motility but works during the interdigestive/fasting phase.

High fibre also increases the time it takes for the stomach to empty. Slow emptying can contribute to blockages known as bezoars. However, dysregulation of the gastric emptying mechanisms, can occur due to an unhealthy gut microbiome.

To wrap this section up, we can see that:

- Poor muscular function/quality

- A diet too high in fibre (and every individual is different in what they can handle)
- A diet too high in fat for that individual
- Poor Housekeeping function
- Too much snacking on solids which does not allow the interdigestive state that is necessary for the action of motilin
- A poor microbiome
- Poor digestion – insufficient enzymes to break down food
- Poor diet with a lack of nutrients required to make the digestive hormones.

can all contribute to gastroparesis.

This list is not exhaustive by any means but it does begin to show just how complex the digestive system is and some of the events that can impact its optimum working. I have not even included nervous involvement, in the above, either.

Gastroparesis

There are many troubling symptoms associated with connective tissue disorders but the main one that affects quality of life, I am informed, is gastroparesis. Gastroparesis is a symptom that is commonly associated with conditions like multiple sclerosis and Parkinson's disease but the underlying aetiology is likely to be different from that of those with EDS. In multiple sclerosis and Parkinson's disease the villain is generally of nervous origin whereas in EDS it is the quality and/or quantity of its main protein that is the main cause of the problem.

Of course, this isn't the whole story. We cannot say that all gastroparesis found in a condition like multiple sclerosis is entirely due to nervous origin. In a similar vein, we cannot say that all gastroparesis found in EDS is due to poor connective tissue. The many hormonal influences of post-prandial and interdigestive states are not necessarily limited to a condition. Therefore, someone with MS may have gastroparesis due to poor nerve function but that does not mean that a high fat diet, for example, is not contributing to this condition.

The Main Hormones Controlling Gastric Motility and Emptying (revisited)

The rate of gastric emptying is controlled by either nervous or hormonal factors.

There are a number of hormones that control the rate of gastric emptying. Cholecystokinin and gastrin act to relax the proximal stomach and enhance contractions in the pyloric sphincter. Either of these actions could inhibit the movement of food into the small intestine. Secretin also inhibits gastric emptying. However, secretin can be inhibited by H2 antagonists.

There are a number of over the counter H2 antagonists that most people will be acquainted with. The most popular H2 antagonists are:

- Ranitidine (Zantac)
- Cimetidine (Tagamet)
- Nizatidine (Axid)
- Famotidine (Pepsid)

On the other hand, an acidic environment is necessary for good digestion. Vomiting of undigested food hours after it has been eaten is characteristic of gastroparesis.

This characteristic suggests that:

- Digestive enzymes are lacking
- Stomach acid has been compromised
- The pyloric sphincter is not allowing chyme through
- The contractions are too weak to mix the food up with the stomach acid and enzymes
- The small intestine has not emptied itself sufficiently due to poor housekeeping action so that gastric emptying is delayed.

A slowing of gastric motility can occur when glucose, fat or amino acids come into contact with the duodenal mucosa. The produces an inhibitory mechanism that causes a decrease in the pressure of the fundus. This lowered pressure slows down the rate of gastric emptying.

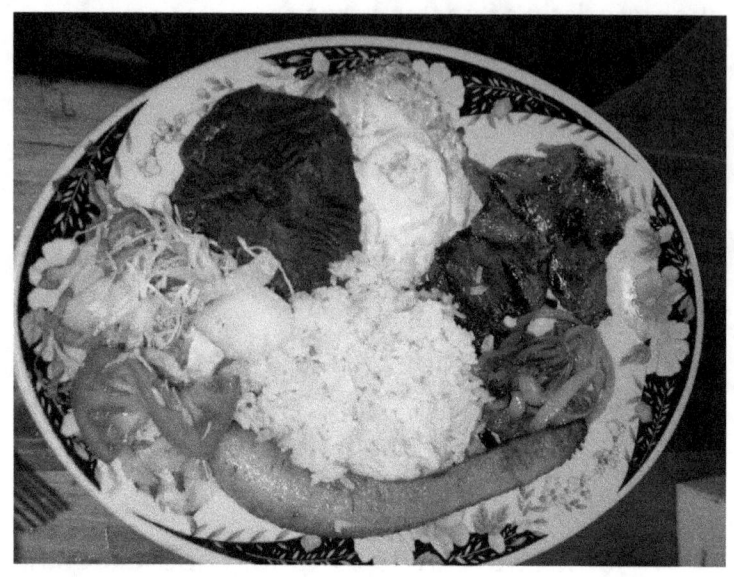

Food in general, can slow down the rate of gastric emptying

How does gastric emptying occur?

- ingested food is crushed, ground and mixed, liquefying it to form what is called *chyme*.

- chyme is forced through the pyloric canal into the small intestine, a process called gastric emptying.

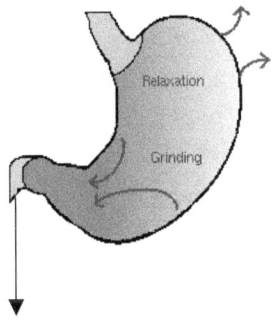

Relaxation

Grinding

To small intestine

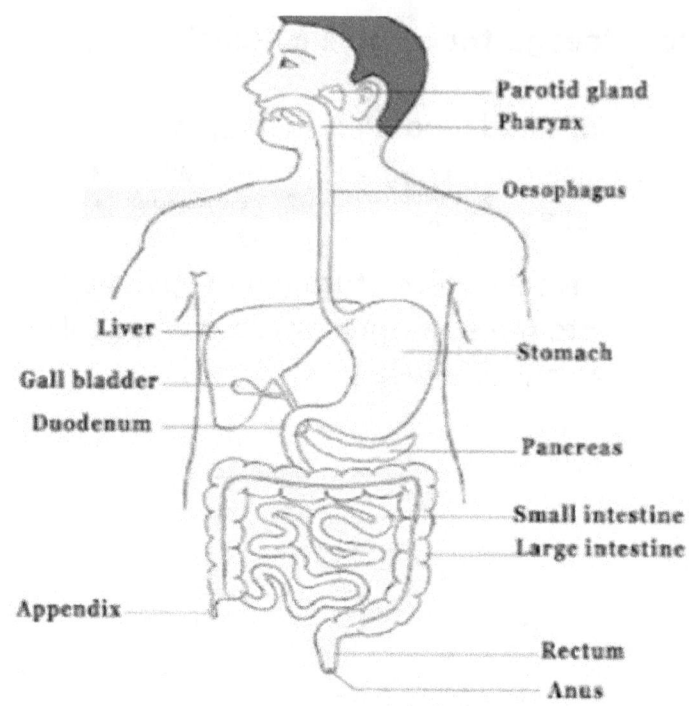

The two other main hormones that stimulate gastric emptying are:

- Somastatin
- Motilin

Somastatin's mode of action is due to its ability to inhibit regular peptides that slow down the action of gastric emptying. Motilin has direct effects on gastric emptying. It is to this hormone that we shall now turn so that we can look at it in more detail.

Motilin

Motilin is also known as the 'Housekeeper of the Gut' as it improves peristalsis in the small intestine helping to clear out the gut to prepare for the next meal.

It consists of a large molecule containing many amino acids.

Motilin needs an alkaline pH in the duodenum. This has a stimulating effect on peristalsis. This hormone has been used off label for gastroparesis.

Motilin, unlike many other hormones that regulate gut motility, is released in the interdigestive or fasting state.

Amino acids in Motilin

Phenylananine valine proline isoleucine tyrosine glycine glutamic acid leucine glutamine arginine   methionine lysine aspartame

Glucose is known to inhibit the release of motilin. Therefore, individuals on a diet consisting of mainly simple carbohydrates will find that their rate of gastric emptying may be inhibited.

Simple carbohydrates include:

The contractions that motilin induce are identified as hunger signals. An antibiotic, erythromycin, can fit into receptor sites found on the molecule motilin. It has been found to stimulate hunger and food intake. It is well known for loosening the bowels when it is taken.

In spite of helping to empty the small intestine, Motilin increases hunger in preparation for the next meal. You can see how - when there has been an overnight fast - most people open their bowels first thing in the morning before 'breaking their fast.' This is motilin's influence.

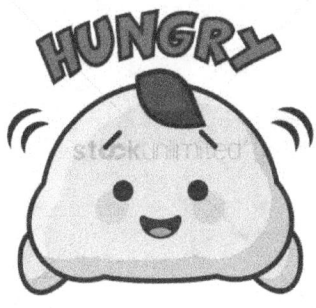

2

Motilin influences these actions through a cholinergic pathway. This means it uses a substance called acetylcholine to send its messages.

Acetylcholine is a substance that is required throughout the brain. One of its functions is to help muscles contract such as that found in gastric motility. We shall come back to acetylcholine later.

As we have seen motilin stimulates contractile activity in the stomach and small intestine. However, the hunger hormone, ghrelin, can accelerate gastric emptying, too. It appears to

---

² https://www.stockunlimited.com/vector-illustration/cartoon-character-hungry_1957190.html

be able to cross react with the receptors on motilin.

PERISTALSIS

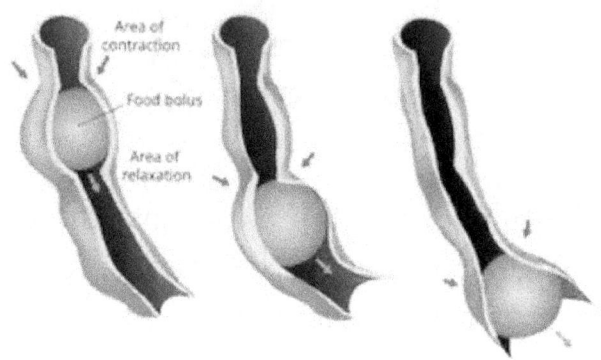

[3] motilin and ghrelin stimulate peristalsis

Acetylcholine

As we have already seen, the neurotransmitter is extremely important in helping muscles to contract. These include the muscles used for peristalsis. One of the main macronutrients required to make acetylcholine is choline.

---

[3] https://www.shutterstock.com/search/peristalsis

The Macronutrient Choline

Choline is a recently discovered macronutrient which has some similarities with the Vitamin B complex. Both support brain and body function. It has numerous important roles in the body - functions which are carried out repeatedly on a daily basis. These include

- Optimum liver function
- Normal brain development and
- nerve function (nerve signalling) as it is a component of acetylcholine – a neurotransmitter - which helps nerves to communicate and muscles to move
- Healthy metabolism
- Supporting energy levels
- It is involved in methylation which is used to create DNA
- It is used in detoxification
- Increases gastric emptying

Choline is a structural component of fat and is found in foods which contain natural fats. However, it is a water soluble macronutrient.

Small amounts of choline are made in the liver but these small amounts are not nearly enough to make up what is considered to be the acceptable intake.

Choline and the neurotransmitter acetylcholine are both involved in a rechargeable chemical cycle. As an impulse reaches a motor end plate the nerve ending releases acetylcholine which instigates events in the muscle cell.

When the muscle contracts another substance called cholinesterase begins breaking down the accumulated acetylcholine and clearing it away. This allows for the next arriving nerve impulse to set the cycle in motion again.

There are approximately one thousand single impulses a second which could not take place without adequate amounts of choline. As choline is generally found in foods which contain natural fats it can be seen that our love affair with very low fat or no fat diets is not conducive to good brain function.

I should underline 'natural fats.' These are fats such as lard, dripping and butter. Indeed, most fats that we have taken out of our diet and replaced with seed oils.

Dietary sources of choline and acceptable intake

As choline has only recently been discovered, a recommended dietary allowance has not been established. However, an agreed acceptable intake is approximately 450-550 mg daily.

Choline is found naturally in cauliflower, broccoli, Brussels sprouts, salmon, eggs, liver, beef and breast milk. Many of these are 'banned' in the low fibre diets those with gastroparesis are advised to follow.

Table 1

Some food sources of choline

Food	Mg per Serving
Beef liver 3 ounces	360mg
One large egg	145mg
Braised beef 3 ounces	117mg
Chicken breast 3 ounces	77mg
Cod 3 ounces	71mg
One large baked potato	57mg
Soybeans half a cup	110mg
Kidney beans	45mg
One cup milk	43mg
Half a cup of dried, roasted peanuts	24mg

Other foods – mainly vegetables – contain smaller amounts of this macronutrient. As you can appreciate, a 'typical' diet is unlikely to contain the Acceptable Daily Intake especially if eggs have been removed in an effort – however mistakenly - to maintain a heart healthy diet. Further, liver is not a popular food now, yet it contains a wealth of nutrients essential for brain health including, more or less, all the choline required daily, in one small portion.

It may be worth jotting down what you eat over one day to ascertain whether the diet provides anywhere near the Acceptable Intake of 450-550mg of choline daily. Fortunately, where tastes, or lack of appetite, mean that the Acceptable Intake is unlikely to be consistently reached, this macronutrient can be obtained at all good health food stores.

Monounsaturated fats help promote a healthy blood flow to the brain. They help to produce and release acetylcholine which is essential for learning and memory; the loss of acetylcholine will result in memory problems often associated with Alzheimer's disease.

Good sources of monounsaturated fatty acids are:

- Avocados
- Almonds
- Cashews
- Peanuts
- Sesame seeds
- Olive oil

Olive stimulates bile which helps the peristaltic action.

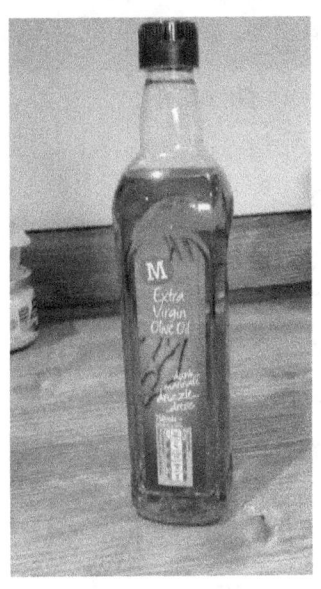

Digestive connective tissue is vital for the regular, but passive, automatic movements in the digestive tract that help propel food along. If dysregulation occurs due to any number of reasons, then symptoms can arise. Some symptoms are gastroparesis or delayed gastric emptying.

Signs and symptoms of gastroparesis include:

- acid reflux
- abdominal bloating
- abdominal pain
- vomiting
- nausea
- a feeling of fullness after eating just a small amount
- the presence of undigested food in vomit from food eaten hours earlier

Now I could, if I wanted, address each individual symptom of gastroparesis but I do not intend to do that since we are trying to treat the underlying cause not the arising symptoms. Each symptom may require one or two medicines to treat it. We are then onto dangerous ground since it is unlikely that we should not have some side effects from doing so that may require the prescribing of yet another drug. Just as an example, acid reflux is a very common symptom of gastroparesis and the general response is to prescribe antacids. These may work in the short term but reducing the pH of stomach acid can result in poorly digested food and further bloating and discomfort. Further, the underlying cause is still not addressed.

I know of patients with gastroparesis who seem to 'collect' prescription drugs with their doctor's approval. I don't know if this reflects the medics lack of knowledge, and experience, so everything and anything is thrown at the patient in the hope something will work.

The response that I would like to see is the expectation that an eventual alleviation of symptoms would be achieved through a bespoke diet and the relinquishment of prescription medications as the condition improves.

It is not a rapid recovery. However, slow improvement and recovery do occur provided constant vigilance and knowledge of the condition inform the treatment plan.

For example, if poor collagen synthesis is the problem then every effort must be made to improve this by, for example, including collagen building nutrients into the diet so that the effects that genes exert, are diminished.

Gastroparesis tends not to be a 'standalone' condition. It is generally a symptom of another condition. As such, it may be influenced by a number of factors that impinge on the primary condition.

It may be useful to look at some of the more common causes of gastroparesis found in conditions like EDS and multiple sclerosis. These include:

- iron tablets
- prescription medications
- poor or insufficient collagen
- lack of certain vitamins and minerals

When I have listened to many patients with EDS there is a common recurring theme and that is that the symptoms became problematical in the teen years when judicious nutrition was not high on the list of priorities. One lady I spoke to informed me that her diet was so poor, when she was at university, that she was prescribed vitamin D tablets and iron. She had never recovered from her malnourished state at university nor indeed, felt it necessary to pay heed to her diet. She was later diagnosed with EDS and is now wheelchair bound and tube fed.

Some of the common medications given to people, who are malnourished, are iron and vitamin D. This is also true of those with EDS. Many people who have had children will know that iron tablets are generally required during pregnancy. Many mums will testify that the iron tablets caused them to be constipated for the very first time.

Why is iron constipating?

Iron is hard on the digestive tract and frequently causes constipation. It isn't easy to absorb as it needs to have a particular charge to be absorbed by the cells of the small intestine. Iron will only be absorbed in the small intestine if the iron is in its ferrous state. Ferric iron cannot be absorbed so it will travel to the colon where it is likely to cause dysbiosis (imbalance of good and bad bacteria) and subsequently, constipation.

Even when iron is absorbed in the small intestine, it needs to go through a series of reactions before it can be made available to the body.

Slow release forms of iron – which are sometimes prescribed – are not necessarily less constipating. The first part of your intestine – the jejenum and duodenum - are where the iron is absorbed best. However, slow release iron may not be released until it reaches the colon where it has the potential to cause dysbiosis.

The colon is full of bacteria that regulates the gut environment, supports bowel motility and stool quality. In other words, as we have already seen, a healthy gut biome means healthy bowel movements.

Pathogenic gut bacteria feed on iron and can upset the balance of the gut biome. *Constipation suggests that an unhealthy balance of gut bacteria exists in the colon.*

It is always recommended that an iron supplement **isn't** taken when an individual has an acute bacterial infection since the protective effects of the gut biome are compromised.

To reduce the chances of suffering from the side effects of iron, use the lowest dose possible. There are some non-constipating forms of liquid iron available. Ask your doctor to prescribe that if it is required.

Milk, calcium and antacids should not be taken at the same time as iron supplements as it reduces the absorption of iron. Taking iron supplements at the same time as the above will definitely cause the digestive problems that we are trying to avoid.

In addition, many antacids that contain calcium have a constipating effect. If you really need an antacid, then choose one that contains magnesium.

Chocolate contains iron; it is also high in fat. Chocolate is a likely cause of constipation through its ability to   dysregulate gut motility. Further, fat slows down the passage of food through the intestinal tract. This can contribute to the digestive issues that we are trying to avoid.

Remedy

- if iron is required use non constipating forms of liquid iron. Do not take with antacids
- reduce fat in the diet but do not eliminate it as it does help absorb fat soluble vitamins.
- Take a tablespoon of olive oil a day as this helps bowel movements. This can

be used with a tablespoon of vinegar and made into a salad dressing. Vinegar is useful for preventing bloating and helps peristalsis – the movement of food along the gastrointestinal tract. Vinegar also introduces new populations of good gut bacteria into the colon.

- Use a prebiotic such as inulin powder to provide 'food' for gut bacteria. This will aid any bloating, if this is one of the more troubling symptoms of gastroparesis.
- Fermented foods help promote the growth of beneficial probiotics or good bacteria. As such they can help with bloating but they do have mixed results on gastroparesis. Some individuals will benefit from adding fermented foods to their diet and others won't. This would be due to genetic differences. Foods in vinegar, kefir, cheese and yogurt are all examples of fermented foods. However, do not take dairy foods at the same time as iron medication.

Narcotics

The ability of opioids to cause constipation comes through their ability to reduce nervous system activity. They block pain receptors in the body that reduces pain. They also block the sensation of wanting to move the bowels. Further, opioids slow down the function of the central nervous system making the stool a hard dry mass.

Stool softeners and medications which increase gut motility (metoclopramide and domperidone) are generally prescribed for constipation related to opioid use. However, they – especially metoclopramide - have unwanted side effects.

 Narcotics affect the whole length of the gastrointestinal tract. Measures which are taken by those with gastroparesis, to alleviate the condition, may prove useful.

Remedy

To relieve the pain that accompanies EDS, and other conditions, and thus avoid the need for narcotics, 6-10g of glycine can be taken daily. Glycine is a non-essential amino acid with inhibitory properties. It comes in crystalline form and is easily obtained, at a reasonable price, online. It is glycine that forms a major part of collagen. I use glycine for pain relief and I have found that it is far more effective than any other form of commonly prescribed pain relief. Further, it comes without the side effects that often accompany narcotics and NSAID's.

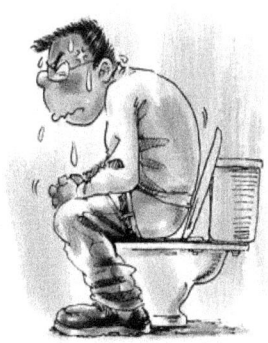

Paul is constipated.

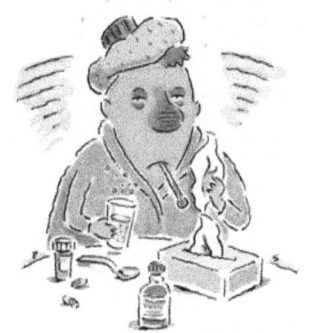

Martin has a cold.
En Martin està constipat.

Other amino acids that have an inhibitory action - and therefore relieve pain - are L-theanine, gamma amino butyric acid (GABA) and adenosine. I will look at these in more detail, later.

L-theanine is found in tea. Brewer's yeast contains good amounts of adenosine which is another inhibitor of pain. In addition, adenosine helps relaxation and natural sleep.

Non-steroidal anti-inflammatory drugs (NSAIDs)

Studies have looked at a range of gastro intestinal symptoms and the prescribing of NSAID treatment for chronic conditions. Popular medications included:

- Aspirin
- Ibuprofen
- Naproxen
- Piroxecam
- Indomethacin and
- Diclofenac

These studies have found that lower bowel symptoms of constipation and straining were far more prevalent in those taking NSAID's than in those who did not take NSAIDs. It was these particular symptoms - more than the dyspepsia that went with NSAID use – which were the reasons why individuals were more likely to stop their medication.

NSAIDs have been found to suppress the contractile activity in the small intestine which precedes the colon. They offer one explanation for the constipating effects of this drug. NSAID's may also reduce the sensation of wanting to empty the bowel.

Remedy

- Use glycine for pain relief instead of NSAID's. Glycine not only alleviates pain but it also has an anti-inflammatory action.
- If a different anti-inflammatory action is required, you can also consider using DMSO which has a powerful anti-inflammatory action. DMSO has to be

99% pure. It must be applied to very clean skin and washed off twenty minutes later. It can be diluted.

DMSO is available online.

- Drink caffeinated coffee. Caffeinated coffee has been found in studies to increase stimulation of the bowel by 60%. This is reduced to 35% in those drinking the decaffeinated variety. Some people would argue that coffee is dehydrating. If this is the case, take a quarter of a glass of water for every cup of coffee that you drink. It is that simple.

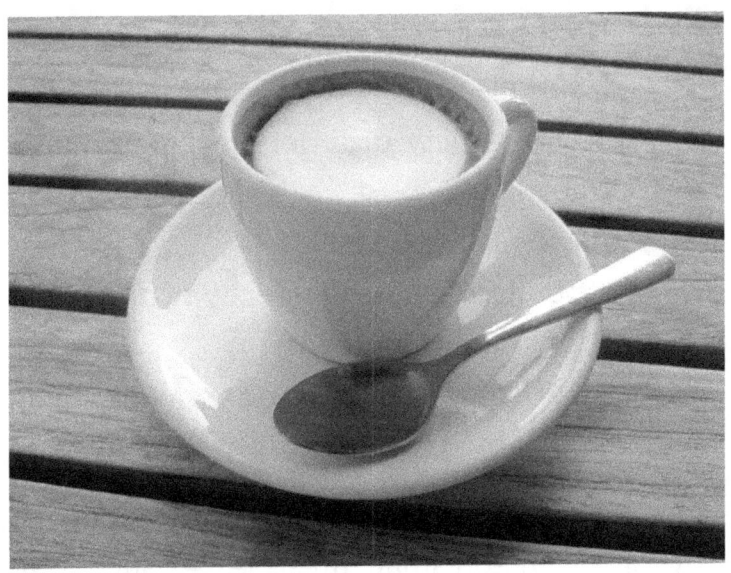

Coffee stimulates peristalsis

The Benefits of Inositol and Pantothenic Acid

Inositol

Inositol is a carbohydrate that occurs naturally in your body and in food. It is a vitamin like substance and is known as vitamin B8. Inositol is used as a treatment for many disorders including:

- Diabetic nerve pain

- Depression, anxiety and panic disorder
- Insomnia
- Some fertility disorders including failure to ovulate
- Alzheimer's disease
- Attention deficit-hyperactivity disorder
- Promoting hair growth
- Treating psoriasis associated with lithium use

Inositol also markedly increases peristalsis of the stomach and small intestine. As such it has a major role to play in disorders of gut motility which contribute to gastroparesis and constipation. Inositol has been used for the treatment of chronic atonic intestine and constipation.

Good sources of inositol are:

- Citrus fruit but not lemons and fruit in general
- Beans,
- Nuts

- Grains
- Bran
- Oats
- Cantaloupe melon.

There is not a Recommended Dietary Allowance for inositol but most diets contain about 1g daily. However, higher doses are used as supplemental treatments. Initially, it is advisable to increase foods in the diet that contain good amounts of inositol but if this is difficult, for whatever reason, then supplements are easy to source online or in good health food stores. Be guided by the recommended dosage on the product label. Inositol does come in powdered form and this is the easier form to add small incremental doses until relief is reached.

Pantothenic acid

Pantothenic acid – also known as vitamin B5 - is a component of coenzyme A which is a substance that helps in the synthesis of choline to acetylcholine. As we have already learned acetylcholine is necessary for peristalsis and it is likely that the increased synthesis of coenzyme A, from pantothenic acid is, responsible for this improved peristalsis.

Good sources of pantothenic acid in food are:

- Animal proteins such as meat, fish, eggs, cheese and milk
- Lentils and legumes
- Green leafy vegetables
- organ meats especially
- Mushrooms

A recommended daily intake for pantothenic acid is 5mg daily for adults. A three ounce serving of lamb's liver would provide 9mg of pantothenic acid.

Six white mushrooms provide approximately 14mg of pantothenic acid.

Pantothenic acid is added to vitamin B complex supplementation which is readily available, at small cost, at supermarkets, in health food stores and online. Most people get enough in their diet but those who chronic illness, poor diets and malabsorption problems may be at risk. It is always worth increasing foods containing pantothenic acid or supplementing if for a short while to ascertain whether this substance can contribute to a healthy functioning digestive tract.

Finally, while vitamin B5 and B8 do help increase peristalsis, nicotinic acid, also known as vitamin B3 has the opposite effect. Nicotinic acid decreases peristalsis in the stomach and small intestine. However, many of the foods that contain pantothenic acid are also the foods that nicotinic acid is found in. It may be useful to buy supplements that are purely pantothenic acid to see if an imbalance in the diet has occurred. Generally, however, the vitamin B complex works synergistically and it is not normally recommended that a supplement of one should be taken to the exclusion of the others.

Antidepressants

Constipation is a very common side effect of tricyclic antidepressants which block the action of the neurotransmitter acetylcholine. When this neurotransmitter is blocked, the muscular contractions which propel waste matter through the digestive tract are reduced. The intestinal secretions which lubricate the intestinal tract are also reduced.

The newer medications like the Selective Serotonin Reuptake inhibitors are less likely to cause these side effects but, nevertheless, may still cause some irregularity in bowel movement.

The idea of blocking acetylcholine is ridiculous. It is this neurotransmitter that is in short supply in those with Alzheimer's disease. It affects memory and learning.

Depression can be either:

- Learned as a reaction to events that appear hopeless.

- Due to an imbalance of chemicals in the brain often induced by stressful events or poor diet.

Remedy

- Talking through problems with a trusted person is helpful for some people.
- Use glycine. Glycine alleviates anxiety.
- Caffeinated coffee stimulates peristalsis that has been compromised by the disruption of acetylcholine.
- The amino acid tyrosine is a precursor for dopamine, a neurotransmitter which lifts mood. Dopamine is in short supply in some people with certain neurological conditions and this is associated with constipation.

Excellent sources of tyrosine are:

- Chicken, turkey and fish
- Dairy foods
- Peanuts, almonds and seeds
- Bananas
- Lima beans

- avocados

Supplemental tyrosine can be taken following the instructions on the container. It can be obtained from good health food stores and online.

The role of hard and soft water in the manifestation of gastroparesis

I have to be honest here. In all my many years on this earth I have never heard of anyone being asked if they live in a hard water area if they are suffering from poorly functioning bowels.

I must admit that it hadn't crossed my mind all that much until I began to explore the reason why bowel habits changed when people moved out of one area into another. Sometimes those snippets of conversations that one hears briefly can make you stop and think. Why do certain things happen in certain places and not others? Do we ever stop and think about environmental factors and the impact that they have on us?

I noticed that when I visited maternal relatives that I suffered from fewer stomach problems, including bloating. I could rationalise it by trying to convince myself that I was more relaxed when I was on holiday but it was more than this. It was only when I stopped over at the part of the country my relatives in and then onto a different area entirely with resultant changes in bowel habits that I began to look into why, more deeply.

I live in a beautiful part of West Yorkshire. The hills are green; the streams are clear. The rainfall is filtered through the limestone, composed of calcium carbonate, that our area is built upon. The water contains calcium carbonate??? Ah yes! Calcium carbonate, the substance that constricts the bowel and causes gastroparesis and constipation.

The presence of calcium carbonate in water qualifies it to be hard water but so does magnesium. Magnesium has a loosening effect on the bowel so your bowel habits may be very much tied in with the area that you live in. Hard water is simply defined by the amount of minerals in the water. The hardness of water is measured by parts per million (ppm).

The hard water capital, of the UK, is Ipswich but West Yorkshire, like London, lags not far behind with a rating of hard to very hard water. This is the highest rating. I know this because there is a very helpful map which shows how soft or hard the water is in the UK.

I have snipped part of the map of the UK to demonstrate how the hard and soft water is distributed.

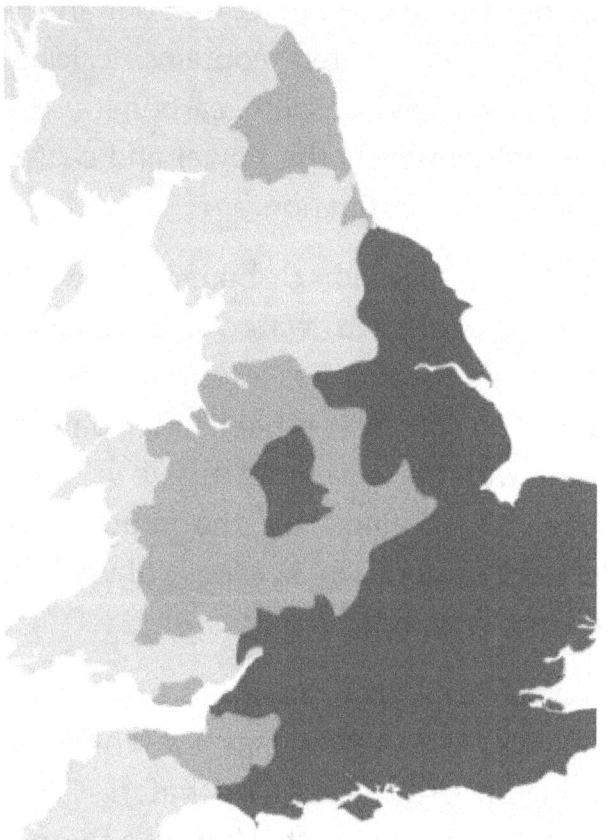

4

The very dark areas are hard water areas. The very light areas are the soft water areas. I live in the area just diagonally above that very dark 'island' in the centre of the map.

There are many areas in the UK that have very soft water. One of the better known areas, outside the UK, are the Dolomites. Soft water does not contain minerals, like calcium or magnesium, in like any of the quantities found in hard water. Scaling of domestic appliances is less likely to happen in soft water areas. Soap lathers so much better. There is less likely to be any adverse impact on bowel habits.

The point that needs to be underlined though, is that the environment impacts on our physical health in ways we do not always think about or understand. Physical problems may not be due to any illness or weakness within us, but a response to prevailing conditions in our environment. We do not always need to take

---

[4] https://www.aquacure.co.uk/

medication; sometimes we just need to skew our diet so that our mineral intake is better balanced. Sometimes that is all it takes.

Table showing how hard water is measured

PPM	WATER HARDNESS
0 – 50 PPM	Is soft.
51 – 100PPM	Is moderately soft.
101 – 150PPM	Is slightly hard.
151 – 200PPM	Is moderately hard.
201 – 275 PPM	Is hard.
276 – 350 PPM	Is very hard.
350 + PPM	Is aggressively hard.

As a precautionary measure if you live in a hard water area - that is built on limestone composed of calcium carbonate - and have gastroparesis or constipation, then consider increasing the foods that contain magnesium in the diet. Supplementation of magnesium may also be considered. In addition , consider filtering your drinking water.

It is always worth noting whether bowel habits change, when you are on holiday, and whether this relates to the hardness, or softness, of the drinking water.

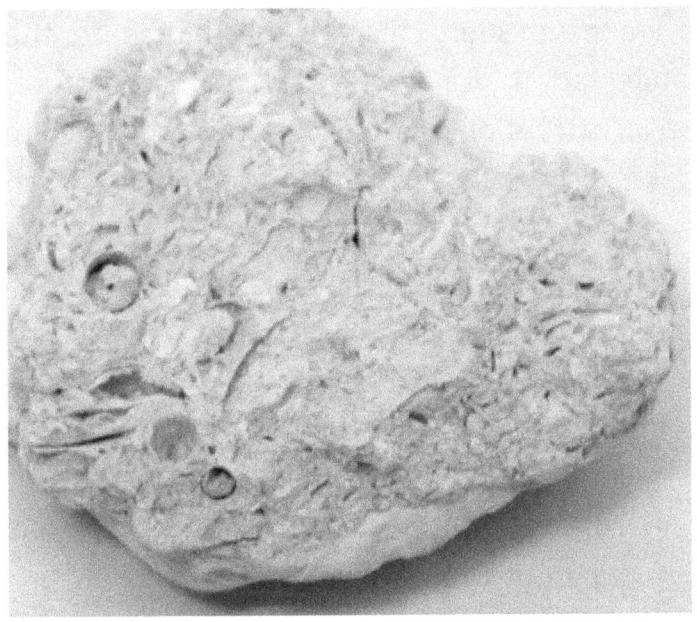

Drinking water, when filtered through limestone composed of calcium carbonate, becomes hard. These minerals constrict the bowel and cause constipation and gastroparesis.

This also leads us to consider whether a diet in foods containing calcium may also be contributing to gastroparesis and constipation. I hear a great deal about how we need to increase foods containing calcium in our diet to avoid the promoting healthy bones as calcium.

As we have seen calcium contributes to the manifestation of constipation. Therefore, special attention should be paid to calcium intake especially in relation to how much magnesium is in the diet.

Good sources of calcium are:

- cheeses
- yogurt
- sardines
- canned salmon
- whey protein (often found in protein shakes)
- lentils
- beans
- almonds
- calcium is also added to flour in the UK

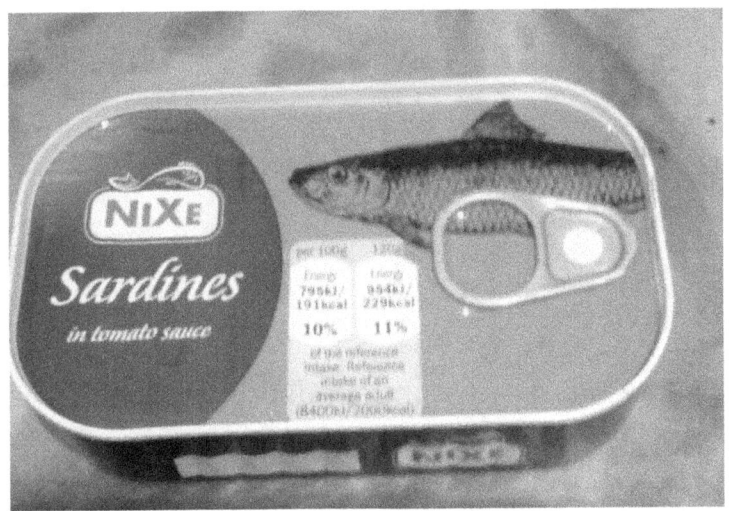

Sardines are a good source of calcium but too much calcium – or an imbalance of calcium to magnesium – may cause gastroparesis

Other unwanted side effects of calcium include:

- muscle pain
- abdominal pain
- kidney stones
- mood disorders

Intrinsic connective tissue disorders causing peristalsis

Remedy

Follow the diet recommended in the book The EDS and Hypermobility Syndrome Diet[5]

---

[5] https://www.amazon.co.uk/dp/B07NBFM1ST

Dysautonomia

The autonomic nervous system controls the bodily functions that we are not aware of such as heart rate and digestive functions.

There are two parts to the ANS, the sympathetic and parasympathetic system. The sympathetic system increases heart rate, breathing and increased blood flow to muscles. In a nutshell, it assists the fight response in the fight or flight reaction to perceived threatening situations. In contrast the parasympathetic nervous system is the 'quiet' sibling of the two. It helps control the digestive system and also prepares us for rest.

Normally, the two systems balance each other out. However, for individuals who suffer from dysautonomia one or the other system will dominate producing an imbalance. This can result in a diversity of symptoms[6] which include gastrointestinal symptoms.

People with dysautonomia look quite well and often experience years of not being believed about symptoms which can be very debilitating. These symptoms appear fleeting and are unpredictable and there is lack of understanding of the impact it has on lives.

Remedy

Check that you are following the diet that would help your primary condition. Include the vitamins and minerals mentioned in this book. A deficiency of vitamin B12 can result in numbness and tingling. However, anxiety can also result in similar symptoms so glycine containing sweets - such as gums -will act as a tranquilising agent.

Make sure that you eat regularly in order to avoid drops in blood sugar which can be

---

[6] Aches and pains, fainting spells, anxiety, tachycardia, hypotension, sweating, dizziness, numbness and tingling, depression

responsible for many of the symptoms experienced by those with dysautonomia. Carry five or six wine gums or other gelatinous confectionary with you. The glycine in the gelatine helps balance blood sugar levels, too.

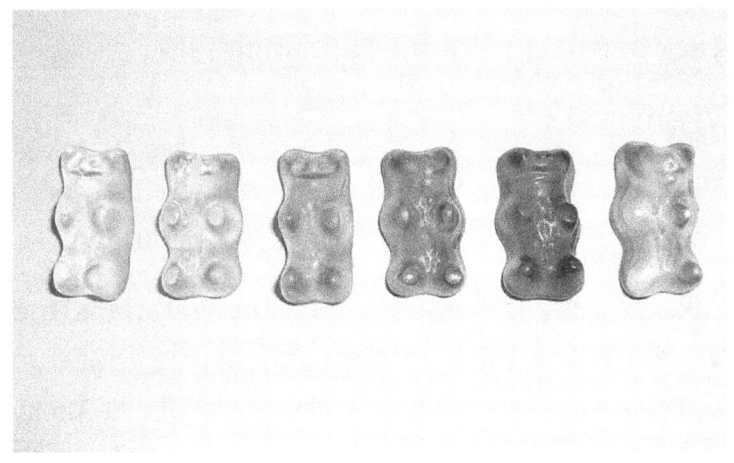

Lack of certain vitamins and minerals

Vitamin B12

Vitamin B12 deficiency is associated with constipation although this fact is little known.

Vitamin B12 is likely to occur in vegetarians and vegans since the vitamin can only be found in animal sources. Meat eaters, who are picky eaters, are also at risk. Those with low stomach acid or who are taking antacids - as many with EDS do for reflux – have an increased risk for vitamin B12 deficiency. An acid environment is required to separate this vitamin from its source and antacids, of course, reduce the acidity in the stomach. This compromises the absorption of this vitamin.

Good sources of vitamin B12 are the organ meats, especially liver. Many people do not eat organ meats as often they were eaten during the 1940's and 1950's. This is a pity as they also contain our friend, the amino acid, glycine.

Vitamin B12 can be found in sublingual form so that it is released straight into the blood stream and bypasses the stomach. This is useful for those with low stomach acid or have poor absorption, for whatever reason.

Vitamin C

Vitamin C is well known for helping bowels move along. When vitamin C is ingested in greater amounts than is required, it has an osmotic effect in your digestive tract. This means it attracts water into your intestines which helps soften stool. When this osmotic stage is reached it is known as 'bowel tolerance.'

However, vitamin C has exhibited a remarkable beneficial effect on gastric emptying dysfunction in diabetic rats.[7] This was brought about by the attenuation of oxidative stress. In addition, the maintenance of the cholinergic contractile responses in the fundus and pylorus were noted.

Interestingly, previously studies have demonstrated that oxidative stress is involved in its onset and development.

Vitamin C is found in all fresh fruit and vegetables. Vitamin C is easily destroyed by heat and light so food should be stored in a cool, dark place and eaten as soon as possible.

It is important to get the right dose of vitamin C. This would differ from individual to individual and is largely dependent on environmental influences. For example, the daily dose of vitamin C was originally set at 30mg which was intended prevent scurvy. However, much larger doses of vitamin C are required for other functions in the body. At 6g, vitamin C acts

---

[7] https://www.ncbi.nlm.nih.gov/pubmed/28639130

therapeutically as an effective antibiotic for respiratory infections.

At lower, but still high doses, it can move bowels very effectively. For some people this 'bowel tolerance' may occur at 1g (1000mg) while yet others may ingest 4 or 5 grams before the watery flushing occurs which empties the bowel rapidly and offers much relief to those with gastroparesis.

It is judicious to take the vitamin C in increments of 1g every half hour until bowel tolerance is reached. The amounts taken should be recorded because you will need to know how much to take daily which is slightly less than bowel tolerance. That is, a dose which helps move bowel contents along without the rapid flushing.

Most people tolerate vitamin C in supplement form very well but some may find the acidic quality a little harsh on their stomachs. In that case the best form of vitamin C to take is buffered vitamin C powder in the form of calcium ascorbate. The amount of vitamin C will be found on the label of whichever brand you choose. Just make sure you take one gram every half hour until a result is obtained.

There are other buffered vitamin C powders – sodium ascorbate generally tends to be cheaper but my preferred buffered vitamin C is calcium ascorbate.

There are lots of different brands out there and which one you choose will depend on your pocket and preferences.

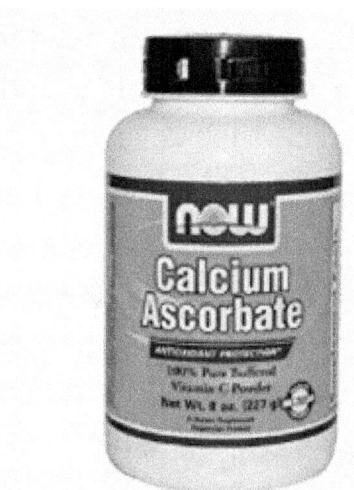

Now Foods Pure, Buffered
Calcium Ascorbate, 227g

You will find that different brands have differing amounts of vitamin C and calcium in them. Some for example, will have 90% ascorbic acid and 10% calcium in them. Others may offer a 50/50 product which means you will require more of the product to get the effect that you want. This can work out to be expensive so a purchase may depend on a number of considerations.

The wonderful part about vitamin C is that overdosing cannot happen. The body will just flush away any excess, rapidly.

During times of stress the body will use up vitamin C rapidly so optimum daily doses can differ from day to day.

Smoking uses up approximately 30mg for each cigarette smoked so a 20 a day smoker is already using up six times the recommended daily amount.

Any infection will use up huge amounts too, so any injury or infection should be addressed using a high dosage of vitamin C.

Vitamin C also relieves pain so has much to commend it for those with gastroparesis

Vitamin D

Low levels of vitamin D have been found to be a risk factor for gastroparesis. Good sources of vitamin D are not in abundance and supplementation is often necessary. However, supplementation should always be taken with a little fat. Vitamin D is a fat soluble vitamin and cannot be absorbed unless a little fat is present. Taking a supplement with a little butter on toast or full fat milk in a cup of coffee will greatly enhance absorption.

You should be aiming for 2000 IU's daily. Vitamin D is obtained from the action of the sunlight on the skin but from the months of October until May, the strength and angle of the sun's rays are not sufficient to synthesise vitamin D.

There are over the counter tests for vitamin D. Some tests only tell you whether you are sufficient or insufficient in vitamin D. They hold little use as their sufficiency starts at 30 nmol/l which I believe is far too low for good health. Optimum levels are between 7—100nmol/l.

There are some tests which have useful reference bandings as a guide on whether to increase your vitamin D3 through supplementation or not.

Vitamin D3 (cholecalciferol) is the active form of this vitamin. There is an inactive form known as ergocalciferol which needs to go through some stages before it is converted to the active form.

For most people this will not be a problem but those with gastroparesis have probably not eaten well for a long time given the discomfort that it brings and may be lacking in trace substances necessary for the conversion process.

Not everyone responds to vitamin D supplementation either and are referred to as 'non-responders.' In this case the addition of supplemental boron in the region of 3- 6 mg will aid this process.

Boron is found abundantly in fruit and vegetables.

Good sources of vitamin D are:

- mackerel and other oily fish
- egg yolks
- liver
- irradiated mushrooms (vitamin D2 only)

Magnesium

Magnesium is a mineral that is well known for its constipation relieving effects. It may relieve gastroparesis if it is caused by a mineral imbalance, or spasm, as magnesium has anti-spasmodic properties.

Magnesium draws water into the intestines. It works as an osmotic laxative – in a similar way to vitamin C - and this increase in water stimulates bowel motility. It also helps to soften the stool triggering a bowel movement and helping to make stools easier to pass.

Foods which are rich in magnesium include

- Meat
- Dairy products
- Fish
- Green leafy vegetables
- Wholegrain bread
- Brown rice
- Nuts

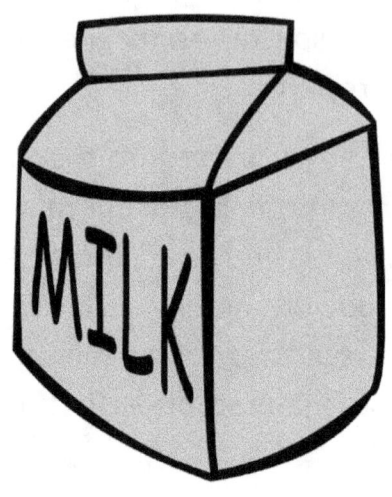

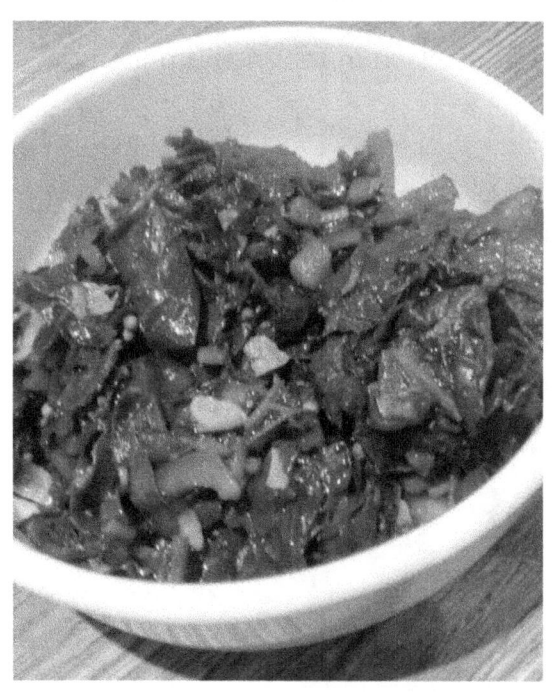

Chard and red pepper dish – full of magnesium

Magnesium is a marvellous mineral which has antispasmodic properties. It is a calming mineral which helps to reduce pain and it is essential for proper muscle function.

400mg supplemental magnesium daily should suffice provided some magnesium is also being taken in through the diet. Some people swear by magnesium oil which can be rubbed into sore muscles. Magnesium can be absorbed through the skin and this effect is taken advantage of in Epsom salts baths.

Many people are deficient in magnesium. As a mineral with over 700 functions in the body, a deficiency needs to be taken more seriously. Certainly, the formulas for those who are tube fed do not appear to contain anywhere near enough magnesium to maintain, never mind promote, health. This should be a cause of concern since sub nutrition will only hasten the progression of the disease when it is not necessary to do so.

Homemade laxative – may help gastroparesis caused by an imbalance of minerals

Caution: the sodium content in the bicarbonate of soda can raise blood pressure so if you have high blood pressure this is not for you

- 1tsp of bicarbonate of soda
- 4000 – 6000mgmg of vitamin C (there are tubes of tablets of vitamin C which make a fizzy drink, these already contain bicarbonate of soda).
- 500mg magnesium (I grind this into a powder but it can be taken separately.

- Drink with some fruit juice which provides potassium.

Mix all together with water and drink. The Epsom salts are bitter and some people cannot tolerate them. In this case omit the Epsom salts and take 400mg of magnesium in tablet form instead.

This can be taken once daily. It can be made up ahead of use and kept in a bottle in a dark place. It can be sipped over the course of the day, if desired.

Pectin powder

Pectin is a soluble fibre found in apples and beetroots. Pectin is rapidly fermented in the gut and forms short chain fatty acids in the process. These pull water into the colon, softening the stool and increasing peristaltic action. If you can't be persuaded to eat one apple or beetroot a day nor incorporate them into cakes or Waldorf salad, then pectin powder is available in health food shops and online. In addition, pectin has the added advantage of increasing good gut bacteria. This will also stimulate peristalsis.

However, in some individuals, pectin can worsen gastroparesis so it is a matter of trial and error.

Olive oil

Olive oil increases peristaltic action and enables the passage of stool that is hard and dry. However, it does not appear to aid gastric emptying directly but it does aid the synthesis of acetylcholine which is required for muscular contractions including those found in the digestive system. Perhaps the role of acetylcholine should be explored further. Choline which is required for its synthesis is in short supply in most people's diets and much more likely to be so for those with chronic illness whose nutritional intake tends to be poor.

We shall now return to the subject of acetylcholine in alleviating gastroparesis as its importance cannot be underlined enough.

The role of acetylcholine in the enteric nervous system

The enteric nervous system is a subdivision of the peripheral nervous system. The peripheral nervous system is subdivided into a further two parts- those parts of your body under your voluntary control and those that are controlled by the brain automatically. The latter we refer to as the autonomic nervous system and it controls and manages responses by your body that we do without thinking including digestion.

The pattern of contractions in the small bowel known as the MMC are controlled by the enteric nervous system. Anything which affects enteric neurons can impact on intestinal movement. As we have seen constipation is very much associated with many conditions such as multiple sclerosis, Ehlers-Danlos Syndrome and ageing to mention but a few. In the ageing process, mechanisms such as the prolonged exposure to free radicals may contribute to constipation. The main neurotransmitters secreted by the enteric nervous system – and also found in the central nervous system – are acetylcholine, serotonin and dopamine. Acetylcholine is an excitatory neurotransmitter and it helps to stimulate smooth muscle contractions, release digestive hormones and secretions and dilate blood vessels. As such, it is required for the propulsion of food along the intestinal tract.

The formation of acetylcholine requires a nutritional substance called choline. Choline is a substance which has only recently been discovered. It has similarities to the vitamin B complex but it is not a vitamin or a mineral. While your body does make some choline most of it has to be obtained from the diet and most people's diets do not contain nearly enough of it. Many people with chronic conditions have poor diets and this, coupled with possible damage to enteric neurons through inflammation, for example, may mean that the production of acetylcholine is reduced below optimum levels resulting in evacuation disorders or constipation. The lack of available acetylcholine has to be considered as a contributory factor in constipation and evacuation disorders over and above the contribution that poorly formed connective tissue and/or any neurological disorders would add.

It is important therefore that the diet contains enough choline to allow for optimum levels of acetylcholine to be synthesised.

A Recommended Daily Allowance has not been established for choline since it is a fairly newly discovered substance. However, an Adequate Intake has been established and this is:

- 425mg for women
- 550mg for men

Some individuals will require less than this and others more. There are a number of groups of people who are likely to require more and, as such be at risk of being deficient in choline. These groups are:

- Anyone with a poor diet or malabsorption problems
- Pregnant mothers
- Nursing mothers
- The elderly
- Vegetarians and vegans

The best sources of choline are foods which are now advised as those that may increase cholesterol levels. As such they are avoided. In addition, the best source of choline – beef liver - has fallen out of popularity. When we take eggs and liver out of the diet then it can be seen that achieving the adequate intake of choline is not easy.

Foods containing choline

- One large egg: 120mg
- Beef liver: one slice contains 280mg
- Salmon: 4 ounces contains 65mg
- Cod: 85gms contains 250mg
- Cauliflower: 120ml contains 25mg
- Broccoli: 120ml contains 24mg
- Brussels sprouts: one cup cooked 65mg
- Soybean oil: one tablespoon contains 47mg
- Peanut butter: one tablespoon 10mg

It can be see that it is considerably harder to obtain adequate intakes of choline in a plant based diet than it is for those who include meat in their meals.

There is no fear in eating eggs. One of choline's functions is to lower cholesterol levels and as eggs contain superb amounts of choline then the hype that they can contribute to heart disease and stroke is unfounded. Choline can also lower blood pressure.

Whenever gastroparesis or any other related intestinal disorder occurs then it makes sense to increase levels of choline in the diet. This is not an overly difficult thing to achieve. For example, stirring a couple of egg yolks into mashed potato before topping a shepherd's pie or making proper Crème Anglaise with egg yolks goes well towards the Adequate Intake of choline. Making a shepherd's pie with minced liver is also a tried and tested recipe in our household. I make this with lamb's liver as the flavour is more delicate than that of beef liver. However, it depends on individual taste. Liver is such a good all round food that it is eaten twice weekly in our house.

If cooking is not your forte, then supplements are useful and easily obtainable online and in health food stores. It is recommended that no more than 600mg of choline is taken daily but be guided by the instructions on the pack.

The next substance that I intend to discuss is the aromatic amino acid L-tryptophan which has amazing bowel moving properties. I think in this respect given its outstanding performance it deserves a chapter all to itself.

Tryptophan

Tryptophan is an essential amino acid which means that your body cannot produce it   so you must obtain it from food.

Tryptophan is required for normal growth in infants. It is also used in the synthesis of many of the body's proteins including serotonin and melatonin as well as niacin which is vitamin B3.

It is required for muscle growth, enzymes which speed up the rate of reactions in the body and the production of neurotransmitters.

The production of serotonin which requires tryptophan also aids sleep and induces a feeling of calm but tryptophan is rarely applauded for its ability to stimulate peristalsis which it does admirably.

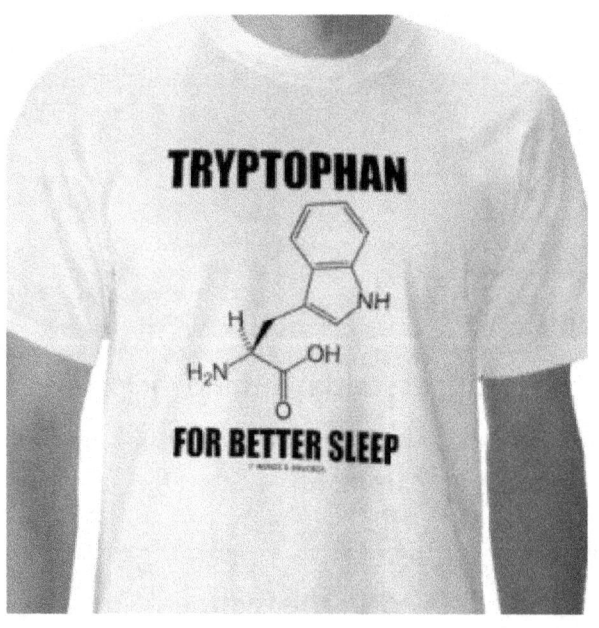

Serotonin is an important neurotransmitter in the central nervous system but also in the enteric system as it regulates motility, the secretory molecules   and the sensibility of the system.

The sensibility is your sensitivity to stimulus which may be low in those with gastroparesis due to a deficiency of the amino acid tryptophan required to make the serotonin.

People with gastroparesis also have low mood, not surprisingly. Tryptophan can address the low mood as well as the gastroparesis

Remarkably, the supplementation of tryptophan at 500mg, half an hour before food 3 times daily and another half an hour prior to retiring can relieve all gastroparesis in less than one day but tryptophan must always be accompanied by 1g of vitamin C daily which can be taken alongside the first dose of the day of the tryptophan.

Both vitamin C and tryptophan are not expensive and may well do away with any other medication or bowel irrigation devices - that have been prescribed - in less than 24 hours.

Tryptophan is found in a wide range of foods including:

Turkey breast

Poultry in general

lentils

canned tuna

oats

nuts and seeds

cheese

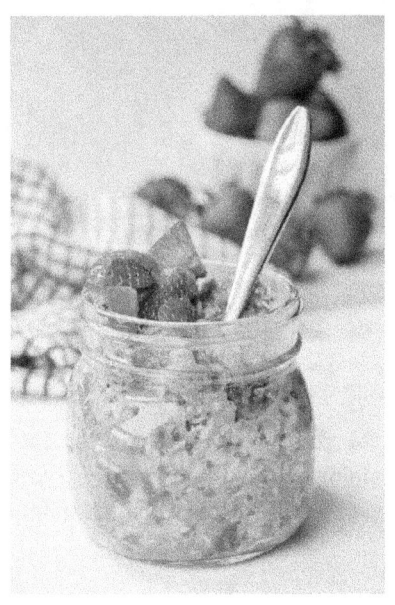

Oats are a good source of tryptophan for vegetarians

By far the best source of tryptophan is whole milk which contains about 750 mg of tryptophan per quart where 500mg of tryptophan is a reasonable amount to aim for, for adults.

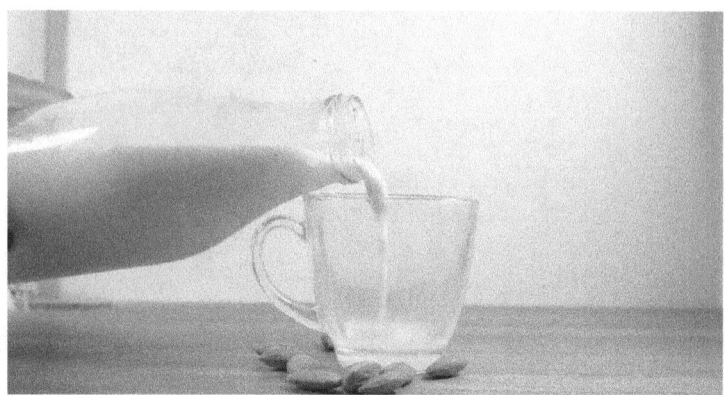

By far the best source of tryptophan is milk. Eaten with oats is a sure way of obtaining excellent amounts of tryptophan which will give you that feel good feeling as well as stimulating gut motility.

As people age, their ability to absorb nutrients declines along with their appetite so that impaired gut motility becomes a probable side effect of ageing by this double whammy.

Laxatives are given to correct this but these medicines are often too harsh and may reduce the amount of potassium and magnesium in the system. The loss of these important substances can actually increase the tendency to gastroparesis so are counter-productive.

Restoring the natural rhythm without the side effects that laxatives bring is the aim which tryptophan and its partner, vitamin C, do more than adequately.

As any effects from taking this combination can be felt within half an hour then the correct dosage can be ascertained in less than a day with proper gut function returning in that time period. It truly is an amazing partnership.

I am now going to turn to other possible causes of gastroparesis which are intertwined with a potential cause for IBS with constipation.

Since the 1940's the addition of numerous nutritional substances to bread has been the practice. One of these substances was calcium carbonate which we know as chalk.

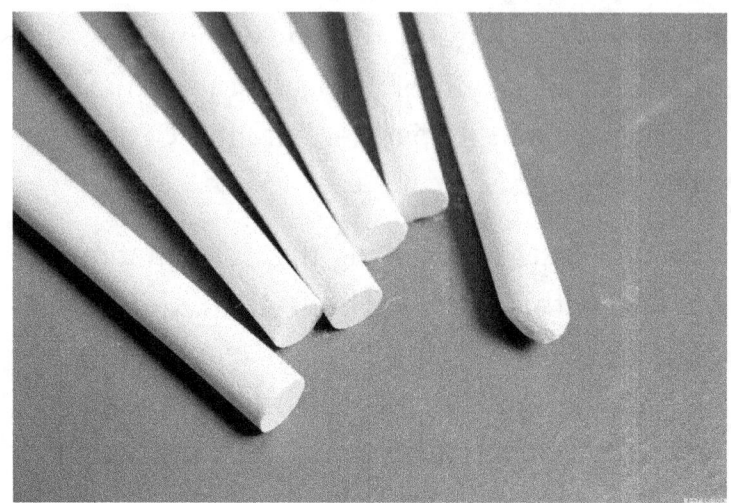

Calcium carbonate is chalk as we know it.

Afterthought – the connection between Irritable bowel syndrome, bread and drinking water.

Irritable bowel syndrome is a new disease. It is often poorly reported due to the embarrassment connected to the symptoms. It is insidious in onset, frequently misdiagnosed and poorly understood.

Prior to the 1970's before formal criteria was gathered to help standardise and define this syndrome, unnecessary surgery was often undertaken to treat IBS. Many of the symptoms of IBS overlap with gastroparesis. Indeed, in some cases they may be one and the same with symptoms differing due only to genetic make-up.

The formal set of criteria was developed in the 1970's after many years of the manifestation of this syndrome.

The mandatory addition of calcium to flour occurred from 1943-1954 to maximise the intake of calcium during a period when food was hard to come by. Many people report thereon to having symptoms of irritable bowel syndrome for which they blame gluten even though tests for this prove negative.

It is quite possible that the calcium added to flour, in conjunction with hard water containing calcium are contributing to this syndrome.

De novo conditions that arise, and impact large sections of the population, are almost always due to environmental factors.

Calcium carbonate is highly indigestible. It requires a highly acidic environment in which to be absorbed. Thus, the elderly whose stomach acid is weaker or those on PPI's or antacids will find that they cannot digest this substance.

Calcium may reduce neuromuscular excitability which will result in constipation as one side effect.

To test whether this may be true in your case use filtered water and flour without added calcium.

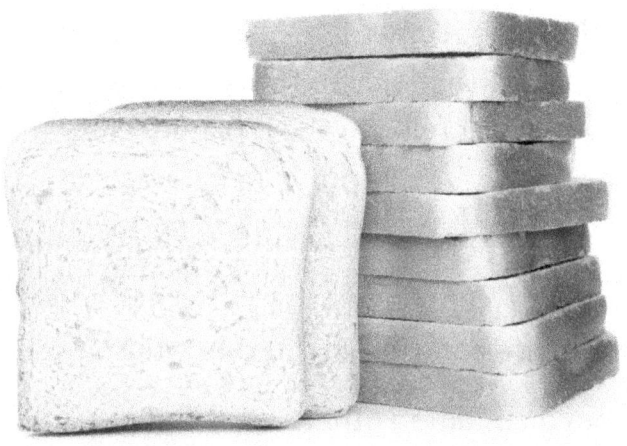

Calcium carbonate is not added to whole wheat flour or bread but fibre may be a problem for those with gastroparesis.

There is another form of calcium which does not have the binding effect of calcium carbonate and further does not need a highly acidic stomach environment to be absorbed.

This form is known as calcium citrate and is far more useful as an additive than calcium carbonate. Further, it is far superior to those chalky calcium supplements that are given to people suspected of having fragile bones.

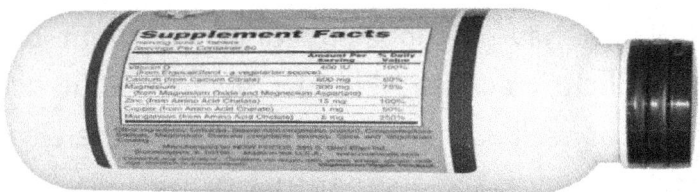

Calcium citrate and useful and absorbable form of calcium.

Citric Acid, Castor Oil, Aloe Vera and benefits of Nitric Oxide

I don't think that any book on gastroparesis or constipation would be complete without investigating the beneficial effects of citric acid.

You may well have come across citric acid before. It is added to some tins of foodstuffs and be included in the list of ingredients as citric acid. In this respect it is just an acidity regulator.

You may find it just labelled as food additive 330.

When purchased separately it is usually in crystal form and has a sharp, sour taste to it as you would find in sucking a lemon.

Tins of tomatoes and tomato juice are most likely to have citric acid added to them but overall citric acid is added to most convenience foods as well as children's sweets. It is the citric acid that gives sweets that sour taste.

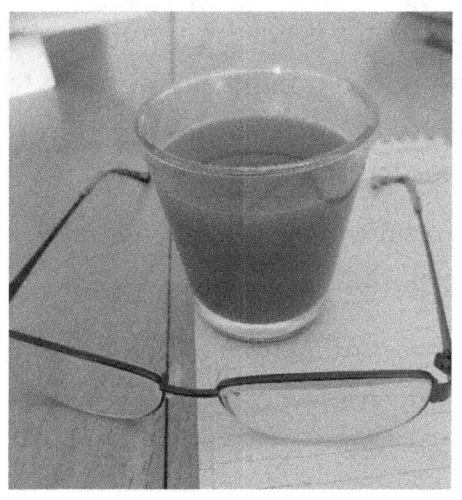

Tomato juice normally contains citric acid.

Acidity regulators are used to change or control the acidity or alkalinity of a food. Changing the pH helps processing, food safety and taste.

They help prevent the growth of bad bacteria and help prevent oxidation that often causes food to go brown.

Citric acid is found naturally in citrus fruits such as limes and lemons as well as the small amount found in tomatoes, too.

The good news is that citric acid is a powerful bowel mover.

Many years ago, it was recommended that you take some hot lemon in the morning to get your bowels moving. People bought bottles of PLJ – pure lemon juice – and followed recommendations but mainly because it was said to be slimming.

It was the hot water, it was stated, that encouraged your bowels to move and the lemon juice was just used as a flavouring or a slimming aid.

I only tried PLJ once. I am not a fan of very tart things and PLJ certainly was just that. It was never described as an acidity regulator or food additive 330 or citric acid.

The very idea that it might help constipation was put to one side. The reality is that it is a much more effective aid for constipation than it ever will be as a slimming aid, that is if you can cope with the sourness.

Citric acid is readily available in supermarkets, pharmacies and online. It is the main ingredient of bath bombs, However, the citric acid that you buy in crystalline form is not the citric acid from citrus fruits. During the war, Italian lemons were in short supply. The importance of citric acid in preservation cannot be ignored, so Aspergillus niger, a mould, was used   as a cell factory for the production of citric acid.

The citric acid produced by Aspergillus niger is the same chemical formula but concerns are around any possible contamination that may occur which could disrupt gut microbiota.

 As citric acid is a stimulant it hurries things along. It is effective so if taken with 300mg of magnesium it can often resolves problems quite easily.

Children ingest far more citric acid than parents probably realise. It is added to fizzy drinks, sherbets and sour sweets. The popular Love Hearts contain citric acid as well as sodium bicarbonate which also increases gut motility as well as reducing an 'acid' stomach.

It is not difficult to incorporate canned tomatoes or juice into the diet. I like making tomato based dishes and soups. Canned tomatoes are also successfully incorporated into breads and fruit cakes and if you want to have a slightly sharper taste then just add a few extra crystals of citric acid or a teaspoon of real lemon juice.

My sister used to make a tomato soup cake. When she first mentioned it I shuddered – tomato soup cake did not sound all that appetising - but when I tasted it, it was probably the best and most moist fruit cake that I had ever tasted.

If all else fails, then a simple glass of tomato juice containing citric acid along with a small slice of those citrusy no flour cakes which use the whole of the citrus fruit is a judicious move for those with gastroparesis.

The addition of a citrus fruit to a cake mix is fairly easy. Take a couple of the fruits, cut a cross in the top but otherwise leave them whole. Add them to a bowl to which you add water half way up the fruit. Microwave for10 minutes. Cut into segments   so that you can remove the pips. Place into a fruit processor and whizz around until creamy. Once this mixture is creamed it can be added to cake mixture. Adding it to almond flour is especially popular.

Citrus dressings for salads are also an option especially if you use olive oil as this also aids gut motility.

Simple citrus salad dressing

Ingredients

2 tablespoons of olive oil

2 tablespoons of citrus juice which can be a mixture such as lemon and lime

½- 1 teaspoon of sugar to taste or a little honey

2 teaspoons of mustard of your choice although Dijon is generally preferred

A little black pepper

Method

Whisk all together and serve immediately

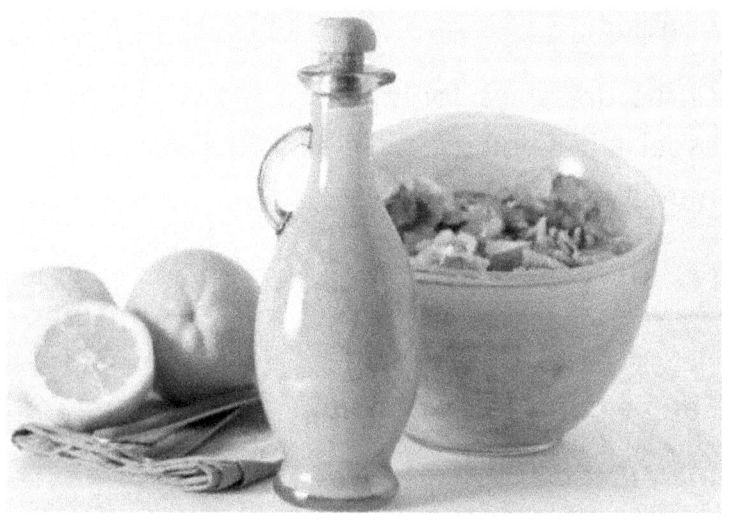

Citrus salad dressing aids gut motility

Although you can do your own investigating by reading labels to see if they contain citric acid, not everyone enjoys this so I have included a list of the more common foods, which are likely to contain citric acid, below.

Foods which generally contain added citric acid include:

- Most soft drinks
- Jams and fruit preserves which also includes fruit yogurts and similar. The more savoury types of food which need an acidity regulator generally use vinegar
- Most canned tomatoes and tomato juice but some of the organic tomatoes may be citric free.
- Mayonnaise is generally made with lemon juice but some are made with vinegar and would then not contain citric acid.
- Fruit flavour sweets which are fizzy or sour. The sherbet and Love Hearts that I used to love so much when I was a child contain citric acid. Just a reminder that citric acid can rot your teeth fairly quickly

so you need to rinse your mouth after eating foods containing citric acid.

- Ice cream - generally the cheaper brands where citric acid is used as a sort of emulsifier.
- Canned fruit
- Stock cubes and concentrates. Chicken is more likely to contain citric acid but I am not sure of the reason unless it would be too bland without this additive.
- Some crisps but not all brand and not all flavours
- Most convenience foods especially if they have added tomato.

Since sherbet is liked by most people as an occasional treat then I am adding a simple recipe below for it. I used to have sherbet when I was a child in which a piece of liquorice was dipped and sucked until all the sherbet was gone.

More recently the sherbet dab has become equally popular. These are bags in which a small amount of sherbet and a tiny lollipop is to be found which you suck and then dab in the sherbet.

The only caution is that sherbet erodes the enamel off the teeth very quickly. It is not a treat that you should be eating throughout the day without rinsing your teeth thoroughly.

As a treat for gastroparesis and constipation, however, it does have much merit.

Sherbet

Ingredients

- 1 tsp citric acid
- 2 tbsp icing sugar
- 3 tbsp jelly crystals (any flavour you like)
- 1 tsp baking soda (sodium bicarbonate)
- Mix all together. That's it.

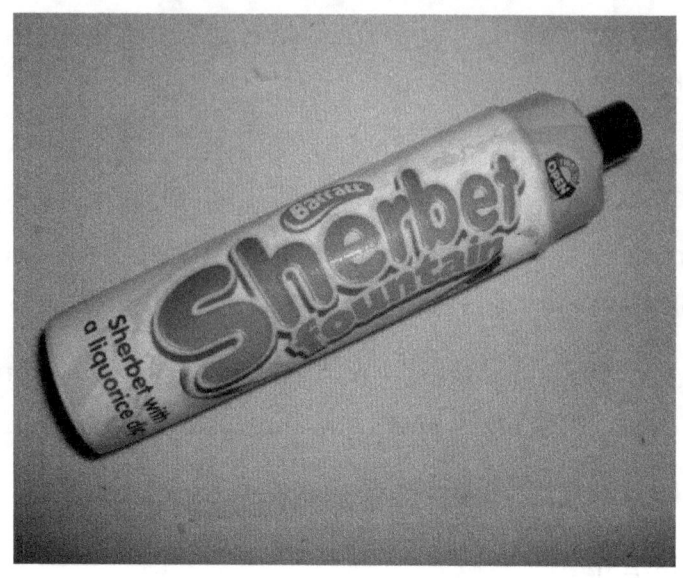

If you take the icing sugar and jelly crystals out
and add 300mg of magnesium you will have
made yourself another bowel preparation which
you can dissolve in water although you may find
that the magnesium comes in tablet form and is
probably best taken that way. Add 500mg of
vitamin C to this mix (it comes in the form of
ascorbic acid and can be obtained in powder

form) then you have made a good bowel mover at very little cost.

Citric acid tends to work very well for most people without any bloating, pain or discomfort that often occurs with other medications designed to assist bowel movements.

With a little bit of thought adding foods containing about 5 grams of citric acid to your diet daily will be helpful for your condition.

However, as you learn which foods contain citric acid you will automatically include them in your diet and benefit from the powerful bowel stimulant that it is.

Many bowel medicines   have been taken off the market recently because of concerning side effects. Once you learn about these common old fashioned responses to reluctant bowels you may wonder why you ever needed prescription medication.

Now, after praising the moving effects of citric acid I need to add a warning about the problems that manufactured citric acid (MCA)

can cause for some susceptible people –
generally those who have food intolerances or
allergies.

 As already stated, prior to 1919, citric acid was
the real deal. It was made from real citrus fruit
– generally lemons imported from Italy. Alas,
like many things, the price of lemons rose and it
became too expensive to add real citric acid to
all the foods, drinks, pharmaceuticals and
cosmetics. Also the logistics involved with
getting the lemons to other countries, including
the UK, during a World War made it imperative
that a different source was found. After all,
citric acid was an important preservative.

After a couple of false starts, it was found that
using molasses and a mould called *Aspergillus
niger*, citric acid could be made and much more
cheaply than importing lemons from Italy.

Given that the synthetic citric acid had the same
chemical formula as real citric acid from citrus

fruits, it was not considered that it would be a problem. However, it was found that many people suffer a diversity of symptoms when they eat any food containing manufactured citric acid. These include symptoms similar to: chronic fatigue syndrome

Fibromyalgia syndrome

arthritis

bloating

swelling

allergic type responses

to name but a few. Therefore, although many people may benefit from citric acid without problem, equally many people will suffer with a wide range of digestive symptoms.

I had half a day looking at the foods in my cupboards. All tomato based products had added MCA (if it says citric acid on the label it will be the manufactured sort). Where real lemon juice is used, it is normally referred to it on the label as lemon juice).

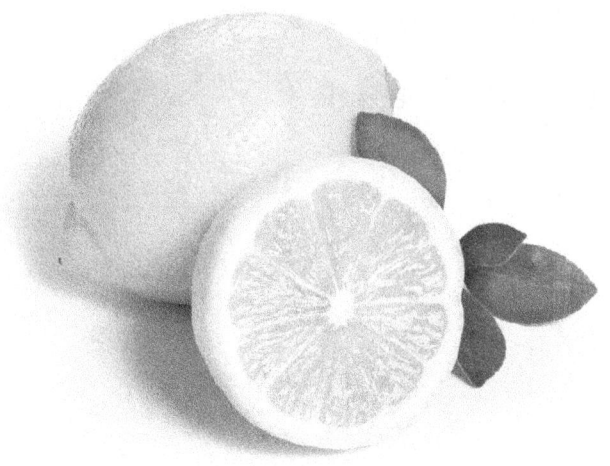

Lemons contain citric acid and give them that characteristic sharp flavour

The tinned fruit that I had in for standby all contained citric acid as did the ice cream, sourdough bread, tinned soup, tonic water and so on. I had some lovely fruity jam - I normally make my own but this is standby in case I run out – and all had citric acid in.

I went on a shopping spree for jam and found all the jams containing real lemon juice cost twice as much even though all the other ingredients stayed the same.

Now, you may be asking yourself why MCA with the same chemical formula as proper citrus fruit citric acid, should cause quite a diversity of symptoms.

It is believed that some contamination occurs and this appears quite plausible. *A. niger* is a mould and even when heat treated is difficult to kill. Even when killed, it can still cause the symptoms that I have described above.

Of course, it does not affect everyone but it worth considering whether to take MCA out of your diet for a few days and replacing it with real citric acid.

Hopefully, for most of the readers of this book, citric acid will be another useful aid in solving some of the more troubling effects of gastroparesis but equally, you may have to take it out of your diet totally. If the latter is the case then there is a lot more work to be done.

Most of your meals will have to be made from scratch. You will find that most of the tinned foods and ready meals will contain MCA.   It can take time to hunt down MCA free foods that you like to keep in.

Sometimes the word citric acid is 'hidden' in some substances. You will find it as a 'citrate' in substances like magnesium citrate or potassium citrate. The citrate is citric acid with extra oxygen.

Magnesium citrate or citric acid are sometimes found in medicines that encourage bowel movements. For example, one of the ingredients in the popular liver salts is citric acid.

Most tonic waters as well as the carbonated drinks contain citric acid. It gives a tart or sour flavour to drink. Elderflower cordial – a wonderfully light and refreshing drink when added to sparkling water - normally contains citric acid.

Elderflower Cordial

Ingredients

5lb of sugar

3 unwaxed lemons

25 elderflowers with stalks, chopped and trimmed (leave elderflowers on a tray for half an hour to allow any bugs to crawl away).

90g of citric acid

Method

To a pan add two and a half pints of water and the sugar. Heat until dissolved then bring to the boil and turn off the heat.

Add the rest of the ingredients and stir well, cover, leave for 24 hours.

Strain and bottle the cordial. Leave in the fridge and when required, add sparkling water or tonic water for a light refreshing tonic.

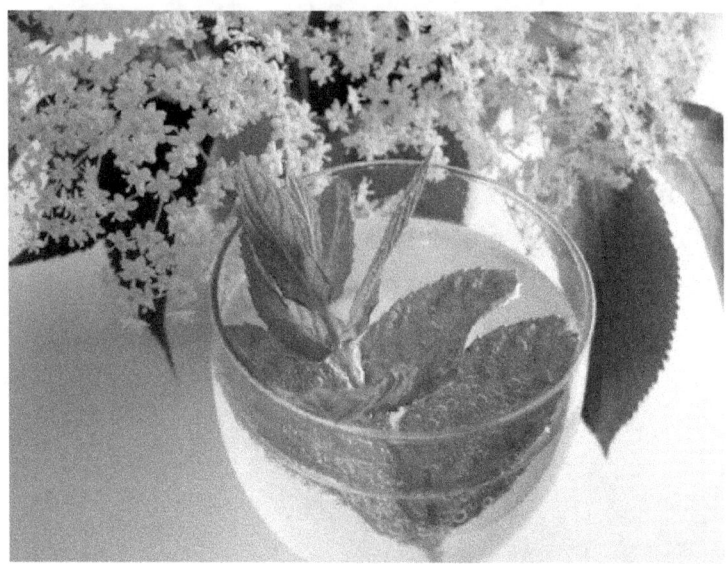

Light refreshing elderflower cordial with sparkling water and a sprig of mint

I find that half a lemon squeezed into sparkling water 'on the rocks' is as good as anything for a refreshing drink. I sometimes add electrolyte salts if I am going out walking on a hot day.

Of course, there is nothing to stop you adding some magnesium sulphate powder for a drink packed with gut moving nutrients. However, magnesium sulphate is a little bitter and you may prefer to take it in the form of capsules.

People can react very differently to a specific ingredient in a medication due to genetic differences as in the case of MCA. Not all ingredients that are added to medications are helpful and can worsen a condition through different pathways.

I have nearly come to the end of this book and have not yet mentioned castor oil. Castor oil used to be a regular favourite remedy when I was a child. It was apparently a cure for all ills. Should there be a hint of delayed bowel movements or even bad behaviour then castor oil was the preferred remedy.

Castor oil has largely been replaced by more 'modern' medications. In fact, many old-fashioned remedies that worked perfectly well for our grandparents have been side-lined for more profitable creations.

The convenient little pills you can carry in your handbag or the salts that address everything from indigestion to constipation are to be found in supermarkets and over the counter at chemists. They are not normally cheap, either.

Now castor oil is used to beautify hair and eyelashes. It has anti-inflammatory properties and can be used topically. Some people with psoriasis swear by castor oil. One elderly lady I know bought some to apply to the dry, flaky skin on her legs and was delighted with the results.

However, castor oil is still good for the gut.

Castor oil is extracted from a castor bean. It contains something called ricinoleic acid which is the main fatty acid found in castor oil.

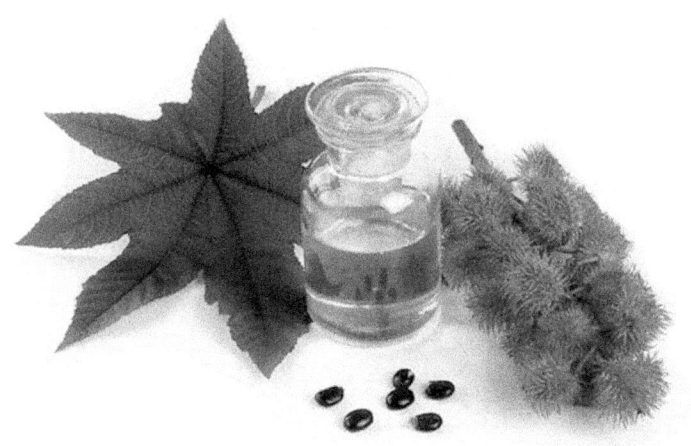

The castor oil bean is full of ricinoleic acid

On the smooth muscle cells found in the intestinal walls there are receptors – tiny shapes that grab onto a specific substance. Once a connection has been made with a specific receptor and a substance then activation of a process begins.

In this case, the receptors we are concerned with are known as EP4 receptors. These receptors are highly expressed in the small intestine and colon. Once ricinoleic acid has attached itself to these receptors, it causes the muscles to begin contracting. In other words, gut motility is increased and the passage of stool is quickened.

Castor oil has more ricinoleic acid in than any other vegetable oil but, unlike other oils, it is not used in cooking due to its petroleum like heavy flavour and gut moving properties.

The normal dose of castor oil is 15ml – three teaspoons - and this may be useful for a first dose. Results are usually obtained in 2-6 hours. You could always try 5mls with each meal on the first day.

After that, reduce it and see how far you can do so before finding a minimum dose that works for you.

Castor oil can also be made into warm packs and placed on the abdomen for 30 minutes or so. This may also induce a bowel movement and get everything going again.

Castor oil has also been useful in cases of inflammation in the stomach known as gastritis. It relieves bloating, reduces pain and straining.

Although there isn't any medication or treatment that is recommended long term for acute conditions, when there is a chronic condition then this has to be managed in the best way possible until the underlying cause is found and dealt with – where that is possible.

Like most medications with a laxative effect there is always the chance that there would be a loss of nutrients - including potassium and magnesium - which are necessary to assist the gut in moving.

As long as you understand this, then you can address any deficiency that may occur – electrolytes really are vital to good health including gut health and movement.

As it is, many people if they don't take castor oil in the gelatin capsules, will add it to a glass of orange juice before swallowing it. This disguises the taste and, of course, the orange juice provides potassium without which, gut motility would cease.

Aloe vera

I used to grow many an aloe vera plant. I was fascinated by the sticky gel that oozed from it and is so prized by the cosmetics industry.

Aloe vera has gut moving properties but this time its effectiveness does not come from ricinoleic acid but from compounds known as anthraquinone glycosides.

Anthraquinone glycosides are compounds that attract water into the bowel. This stimulates gut motility and improves the consistency of those individuals whose stool is hard and like rabbit pellets.

This can often happen with those who do not drink enough or are on diuretics which apparently get rid of excess water. However, all that diuretics tend to do is make you thirsty so that you increase your fluid intake.

 However, the ridding of the alleged excess water through urination also deprives the body of the electrolytes needed to stimulate the digestive tract to move.

It can be understood that lack of gut motility can occur because of a number of, and any combination of, reasons.

Aloe vera is not generally a regular part of anyone's diet so it is good to know that anthraquinone is also found in good amounts in fungi. If you are a mushroom lover, then add them freely to your diet. Where you use mushrooms in salad, remember that olive oil also has some gut moving benefits – especially if you add some lemon juice and make a salad dressing.

However, it may not be as effective as castor oil.

Electrolytes like magnesium also attract water into the bowel but do not contain anthraquinone glycosides. Magnesium ions are poorly absorbed and attract water through an osmotic action.

Osmosis is a process by which molecules of a solvent will pass through a semi-permeable membrane from a less concentrated solution into a more concentrated one.

However, the action of magnesium is not thought to occur as a local effect in the gut. It may help to release hormones such as cholecystokinin or activate nitric acid synthase both of which may be helpful in the fight against gastroparesis.

Cholecystokinin is composed of three syllables which gives us a clue as to its job:

Chole = bile

Cyst = sac

Kinin = move

Cholecystokinin is a peptide hormone found in the gastrointestinal system. It is responsible for stimulating the digestion of protein and fat.

 Nitric oxide synthase is an enzyme. It helps convert the amino acid arginine into citrulline. During this process nitric oxide is produced.

The action of many laxatives is nitric oxide mediated. Therefore, it is wise to eat foods that increase the synthesis of – or help preserve – synthase or nitric oxide.

I have included a table of foods that help with this. Some of them have other beneficial actions in relation to gastroparesis, too.

Table showing food which help to promote nitric oxide.

foods	How
Beets – a favourite this one Green leafy veg – the darker the better	Rich in dietary nitrates which convert to nitric oxide
Garlic	Activates nitric oxide synthase
Watermelon	Good source of citrulline (legumes , soy, chickpeas and meat have lesser amounts)
Dark chocolate, nuts (especially walnuts) and seeds, red wine	Increases levels of nitric oxide significantly

Vitamin C	Increases levels of nitric oxide synthase
Coenzyme Q10	Helps to preserve nitric oxide. Found in organ meats like liver and kidney

You can see that different foods have a slightly different role to play with nitric oxide. Some may activate, preserve or increase nitric oxide, for example.

Clever cooks will by now have realised that red velvet cake which is made with beetroot and dark chocolate has a lot to offer those with gastroparesis. If beets are folded into some ground almonds to replace some of the flour in a cake, then this will raise levels of nitric oxide. A main meal eaten with green leafy veg or added garlic – which will increase levels of nitric oxide - will greatly reduce the burden that a condition like gastroparesis places on you.

Nitric oxide is an unstable molecule so food which promote or contain this molecule need to be eaten little and often.

Nitric oxide supplements can be bought from health food shops but I have found these expensive and perhaps only to be used if the foods which promote nitric oxide are ones that you really do not like and would not be included in your diet.

Beetroot and Chocolate Cake Recipe

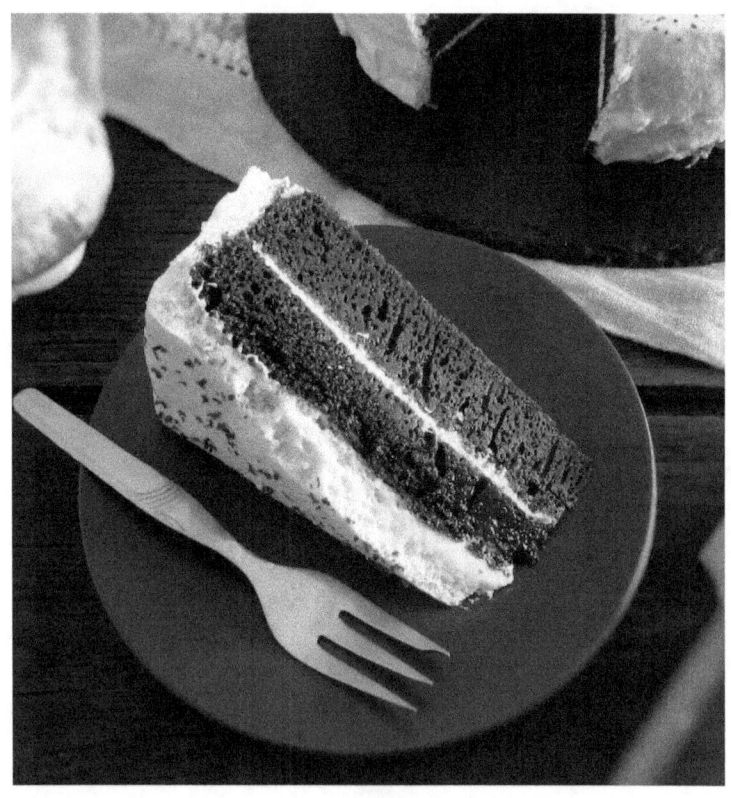

Chocolate beetroot cake is a gut moving delight

Ingredients

200g of cooked beetroot

200g of plain flour

50g of ground almonds or walnuts or a mix of them (optional)

100g of cocoa powder

1 tablespoon of baking powder

200-250g of flour (the beetroot is sweet so use 200g, taste and add more only if needed.)

3 eggs

2 tsp of vanilla extract

200ml of butter or mix of vegetable oil and butter

125g of dark chocolate broken up into pieces

Method

Place all ingredients – apart from the oil and chocolate in a food mixer and blitz until very smooth.

Add oil in a thin stream.

Once you have the mixture blended well, add broken up chocolate to the mix.

Place in a lined loaf tin.

Bake at 190C, gas mark 5, fan 170C for approximately 25 minutes until cooked.

Use a skewer which should come out clean if the cake is cooked.

For me this works well as a replacement meal. It contains loads of protein, butyric acid (in the butter) – which also helps gut function - and many other nutrients for gut health.

Butyric acid is also found in dairy foods like hard cheeses and yogurt so a dollop of yogurt would not go amiss with your beetroot cake.

Butyric acid has anti-inflammatory properties and reduces intestinal inflammation which sometimes causes swelling and impacts the movement of stool through the gut. It also supports the mucosal barrier so 'oils' the gastrointestinal tract and allows easier movement of stool that way.

As people age, the inner lining of their digestive tract can become drier and, may, in some cases, contribute to impaction. Butyric acid – along with castor and olive oil, tend to prevent this from being a problem.

Ordinary wheat flours and grains can also contribute to gastroparesis as we age. Then is the time to stop using grains in cakes and replace with legumes. Most beans do not taste of anything and, if cooked properly and blitzed, make a good addition to the 'body' of a cake.

As well as offering gut stimulating properties, the mix of amino acids found in lentils are kinder on the gut and as they are mainly inhibitory amino acids also anti-anxiety, treat pain and insomnia.

It is quite possible to replace some of the flour in a recipe with mashed beans. I use borlotti beans in chocolate cake (they are cocoa coloured) and the texture of the cake is akin to fudge cake. It is easier to eat and kinder on those with gastrointestinal problems. You cannot taste the beans at all, they just add to the texture.

If I am making fruit cake, then baked beans are a good edition. The tomato sauce goes particularly well with dried fruit giving it a rich fruity flavour as well as enhancing moistness.

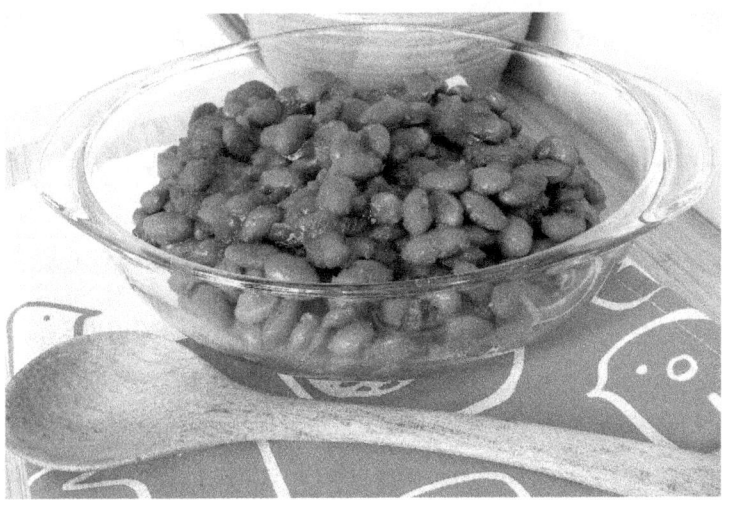

Baked beans are a good addition to a fruit cake if mashed well beforehand.

I will be producing a recipe book for those with gastroparesis in 2023.

Further thoughts

Gastroparesis cases have risen markedly in the last few decades. Some of these cases can be attributed to the rise of diabetes and other medical conditions which are characterised by this troubling condition.

When cases of any condition rise then a judicious examination of likely environmental contributing factors needs to be undertaken.

While most people are aware that opioids are constipating, most people are not aware that NSAID's are too. NSAID's can cause indigestion and the resulting antacids taken can further increase the impact of NSAID's delayed gastric emptying.

It could be argued then, that many of the diseases on the rise are due to the differences in lifestyle and the availability of drugs that can be easily obtained in supermarkets. We can never discount the influence of the environment and our unknowing choices on our health.

It should now be clear that a number of effective remedies are available – other than a low fibre diet - for those with gastroparesis. This medicine chest is easy to put together and has the advantage of putting you in control of your condition.

Further, once you have studied the properties of each remedy you can chop and change treatments depending on which of them appears to be most appropriate or effective at any given time. You become your own detective and begin to have control over the situation.

The importance of a gastroparesis sufferer researching and monitoring their own condition cannot be underlined enough. There is not just one reason that must be addressed, which results in this condition. The digestive tract has never been just a case of food in one end and out of the other and if it goes wrong there is only one reason for it.

The digestive tract is a complex piece of machinery. There are many reasons for it failing to move in the way that we would want it to. One person may find that increasing vitamin C to bowel tolerance is all that is required. Others may find that they need to increase their food intake of foods which synthesise nitric oxide, magnesium and citric acid before relief is obtained. The treatment is as unique as the gastroparesis sufferer.

However, it cannot be said too often – these remedies need to be undertaken alongside a change in eating patterns as has already been described.

I say this for one very good reason. In discussion with many sufferers of gastroparesis, I have found that this condition began when those individuals had volunteered that they had gone through a phase of poor eating habits with poor nutritional intake.

Even when their nutritional intake appeared to be corrected the condition continued. The gut brain connection is important, Maybe, the pattern of abnormal gut motility has embedded itself in the neural pathways as a default position.

If so, then a new default position can be learned but it takes time to do so even for those with no other known underlying disorder.

There are, however, many with underlying disorders which contribute to gastroparesis. Many of these are neurodegenerative conditions such as Multiple Sclerosis or Parkinson's disease which may be amenable to – and require - other interventions in addition to some of the treatments mentioned above.

It may also be necessary to remove – or change - any prescribed medications which are contributing to the condition – and there are many.

I have oft said that a prescription will be issued to deal with one troubling symptom which will then have three or four side effects which the GP hasn't considered but which need further medications to overcome. Unfortunately, many of these side effects do impact gut motility negatively.

Table showing side effects on the digestive system of some common medications

Medication	Side Effects
Paracetamol	May cause liver damage.
Ibuprofen	<ul><li>Suppresses contractile activity in the small intestine</li><li>Damage to mucosa in small intestine</li><li>Alteration in gut biome</li></ul>
Naproxen Sodium	Can cause stomach ulcers and bleeding
Ranitidine	<ul><li>Lowers stomach acid which may increase the risk of infection,</li><li>impairs digestion and the ability of vitamin B12 to be separated from its source</li></ul>

	• Delays gastric emptying
omeprazole	Significantly delays gastric emptying[8]
Aluminium antacids such as Amphojel	Delays gastric emptying
Elavil and other tricyclic antidepressants as they are anticholinergic in character.	Delays gastric emptying
Bulk forming agents like Fybogel	Delays gastric emptying
Diuretics like furosemide can cause electrolyte and metabolic disturbances	Delayed gastric emptying
antihistamines	Delayed gastric emptying
Drugs for neuropathic pain such as	Delayed gastric emptying

[8] https://onlinelibrary.wiley.com/doi/pdf/10.1111/j.1365-2036.2005.02528.x

Pregabalin and Gabapentin	

Enzymes

Right at the beginning of this book I mentioned how food needed to be broken down enough to pass through the pylorus muscle. If food was not broken down enough then gastro emptying would be delayed.

There are a number of reasons why food may not be broken down so that it is unable to pass through this important muscle and we will examine these now.

The first reason will seem obvious. Food needs chewing and chewing well. When I was little and family meals were always taken at the table in a leisurely fashion, then this was not problematical. Indeed, we were told to chew our food a hundred times before swallowing. I thought that this was far too much although I tried it a couple of times but it somehow spoiled my enjoyment of food.

However, family meal times did tend to be less rushed. It was a social meal and could last a considerable length of time. A half hour rushed snack before heading back to work was unheard of.

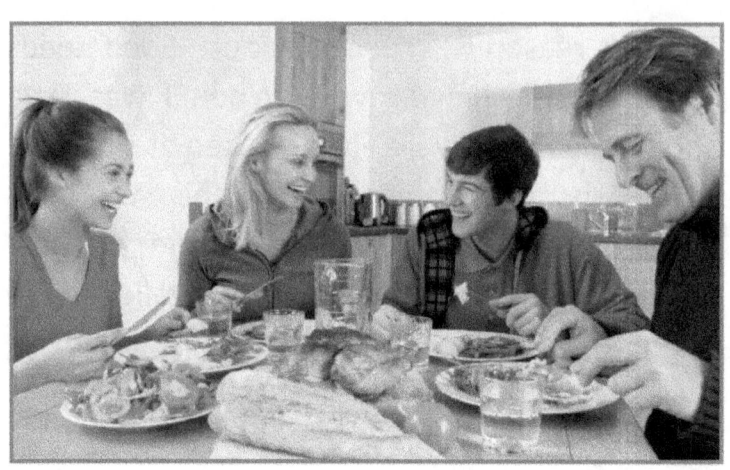

Eating should never be a rushed affair

We were also encouraged to take small bites and lay our fork down again until our mouth was empty.

Although these are small steps the act of chewing and covering in saliva begins the digestive process as well as enabling the bolus of food to slide easily down the oesophagus and into the stomach.

Normally, the stomach is very acidic. It has a pH of around 2 due to the hydrochloric acid that it contains.

The stomach is mainly an area which holds and begins the digestion of proteins.   If the main meal consists mainly of protein, then the food will be held in the stomach for a few hours until the food is broken down completely.

The stomach churns the acid and coats the food with it but clearly if large chunks of protein have been swallowed without much chewing then the whole process is going to take quite long before the contents are small enough to pass through the pylorus muscle.

The acidity activates pepsin which is a protein digesting enzyme. If activated properly it will begin to break down the protein. Eventually, the breakdown of protein will produce a substance known as chyme. This has a porridge like consistency and can easily pass through the pylorus muscle provided there is enough acetylcholine to initiate impulses.

The acid helps activate the pyloric sphincter enabling it to allow chyme through and into the next stage in the small intestine.

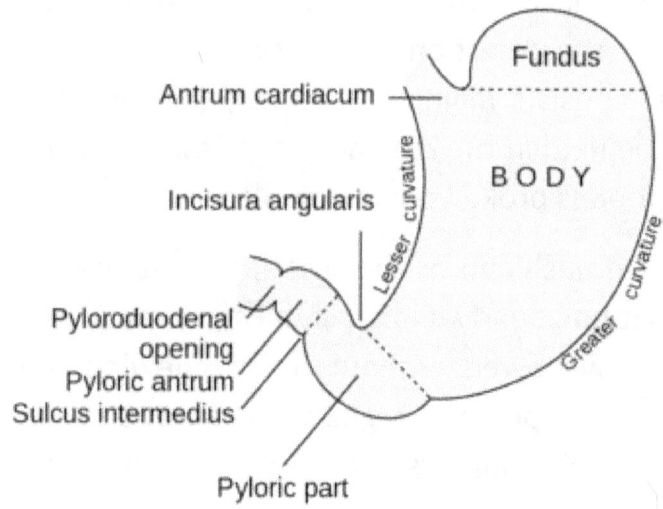

Fundus

Antrum cardiacum

Incisura angularis

Lesser curvature

B O D Y

Greater curvature

Pyloroduodenal opening
Pyloric antrum
Sulcus intermedius

Pyloric part

Any prescribed or over the counter medicine which raises the pH levels towards greater alkalinity will greatly slow down the vital process of the breakdown of protein and its subsequent passage through the pyloric sphincter muscle

Antacids are easily over the counter medicines for indigestion and heartburn. PPI's like Omeprazole and Lansoprazole have become very popular prescriptions but do not come without many negative side effects.

A weakly acidic environment means that many nutrients cannot be absorbed. Vitamin B 12 for example is attached to a protein source and cannot be separated from it   unless there is a sufficiently acidic environment in which to do so.

However, the inability to properly absorb also affects magnesium, calcium zinc, among many others. It is no wonder that osteoporosis is a casualty of older age when stomach acid tends to weaken.

Zinc is responsible for the synthesis of many enzymes and macromolecules. Without it we simply cannot make the necessary chemicals for many of the functions in the body.

The stomach really holds the key to many of the degenerative processes that occur in the body if the acidic environment is tampered with.

The acid environment also destroys pathogens that may have been hiding in the food.

From this we can gather that gastroparesis may be caused by a lowered acidic stomach environment which not only slows down the breakdown of protein into chyme but also fails to activate the pyloric sphincter muscle so that the chyme is not enabled to pass through it.

The stomach will feel very heavy and uncomfortable. Some people will only experience this after a very heavy meal but others experience the bloating and heaviness after even light meals.

One has only to consider that if an individual eats a high protein meal and then takes an antacid or a PPI that they are setting themselves up for trouble. Even milk which is full of goodness – and protein – can be problematical in spite of the fact that it is a liquid.

Many people are quick to blame lactose and pay extra for lactose free milk to try and correct the bloating and discomfort that an intolerance can bring. No-one ever thinks that it may be lack of stomach acid because this is not popular knowledge. We know mainly what we are fed through clever advertising. However, hundreds and thousands of individuals would be far better off stopping the antacids and increasing their stomach acid naturally.

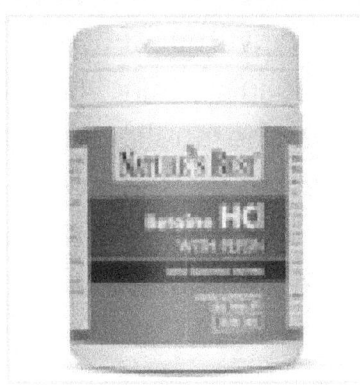

There are hydrochloric acid tablets available as a supplement normally advertised as HCL betaine. They may also contain that digestive enzyme pepsin which is all to the good because ageing also diminishes the production of this important protein digesting enzyme

For the amount of relief, a supplement like this has the potential to give it is worth a try.

Betaine is also known as folate or vitamin B9. It assists in giving the stomach acid levels a boost so that the breakdown of food is effective and quick.

 Betaine can be synthesised within the human body from choline. Choline is needed to synthesise two phospholipids that are integral part of cell membranes. However, choline, In the context of addressing gastroparesis, is need to produce the neurotransmitter acetylcholine the subject of which I introduced in a previous chapter.

Choline is both fat and water soluble. The distinct molecules are transported and absorbed differently. The water soluble forms are converted in the liver to lecithin.

How gastroparesis may occur

Stomach acid
activates pepsin a
protein digesting enzyme
which breaks down
protein into a sludge.

→ Chyme

Chyme can only pass
into the small intestine
through the pyloric
sphincter muscle if:

1) the environment is
strongly acid

2) There is enough
Choline In the diet.
This makes acetylcholine
which causes pyloric
sphincter to contract

Acetylcholine, you may recall is required for the initiation of the muscular contractions which enable chyme to move from the stomach to the small intestine.

Choline is found in a number of foods including:

Poultry

Fish

Red meat

 Dairy products – milk, cheese, yogurt

Eggs

Nuts

Seeds

Whole grains

Cruciferous vegetables like cauliflower

beans

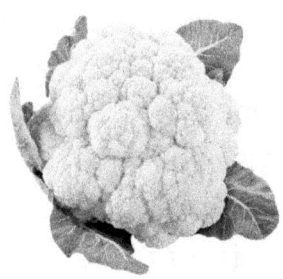

Cauliflowers are a good source of choline

The upper tolerable level for choline can be seen below.

Table 3: Tolerable Upper Intake Levels (ULs) for Choline [2]

Age	Male	Female	Pregnancy	Lactation
Birth to 6 months*				
7–12 months*				
1–3 years	1,000 mg	1,000 mg		
4–8 years	1,000 mg	1,000 mg		
9–13 years	2,000 mg	2,000 mg		
14–18 years	3,000 mg	3,000 mg	3,000 mg	3,000 mg
19+ years	3,500 mg	3,500 mg	3,500 mg	3,500 mg

With beef liver providing 357mg of choline per three ounce serving and one egg providing 148g of choline. These are the two highest sources of choline.

To sum up one of the main causes of gastroparesis may be heavily influenced by environmental considerations given the lack of time individuals devote to eating in a calm and relaxed way. The clock rules now and many people are given very limited meal breaks at their place of work.

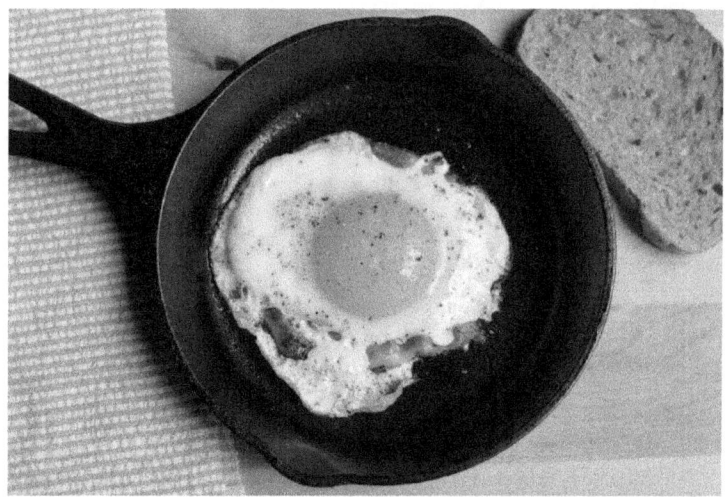

One egg provides 148mg of choline. Eggs are the second highest provider of choline and should be eaten on a regular basis. They are an excellent source of nutrition.

Foods containing protein are eaten more nowadays – the burger 'on the go,' the half pound steak at the funfair which I recently saw advertised, the whey proteins which are so popular all may contribute if the amount of protein an individual is trying to digest outweighs the body's ability to produce pepsin.

Of course, if betaine – which is required to strengthen stomach acid levels – is low then the synthesis of choline is low. If the synthesis of choline is low then the knock on effect is that the neurotransmitter, acetylcholine cannot be made in sufficient quantities. Acetylcholine, of course is required to fuel the muscular contractions of the pyloric sphincter muscle without which the chyme will just sit unable to pass through into the smaller intestine.

Food really is a medicine. If you don't have a well- balanced diet, then many of the nutrients that you require for the millions of functions that are required in the body to keep it ticking over will simply not happen.

A percentage of the royalties from the sale of this book are donated to charities like the one below.

The Exodus Project

My first introduction to the far reaching impact of The Exodus Project occurred when I was travelling around Cawthorne in one of their buses, visiting gardens.   A young lad was happily munching on a sandwich. He looked up briefly, pointed to the driver and said,' He's my second dad, he is,' then he returned to his sandwich without further comment

Such remarks are often very telling and so I arranged to meet Jackie Peel and Martin Sawdon, at the charity's premises in Barnsley. They set up the Exodus Project 20 years ago. They moved into their current premises – a redundant Methodist church - in 2010.

Both Jackie and Martin have been youth workers in their church. Martin worked in housing for the homeless in addition to working in learning disabilities services in institutional settings.

The work that the Exodus Project undertakes is of paramount importance to the communities it serves. These were former mining communities which became disadvantaged after pit-closures. Currently about 400 children attend mid-week activities from Monday to Thursday inclusive. These activities include dance, drama, craft, music, sports and games. In addition, there are weekend camps, cycle treks, outward bound activities, bowling and swimming. The children are taught valuable life skills including how to cook and bake. It is all about teaching children how to fulfil their potential and learn skills they will be able to pass onto the next generation.

The grounds, once overgrown, have been turned into a play- and camping - ground. A miniature railway is in the process of being installed.

Martin and Jackie have developed a unique model in that The Exodus Project goes beyond dispensing services. They are keen to build up relationships with the whole family and not just the child that attends the mid- week clubs. In addition, once children have reached the age of fourteen, they are invited to help out with the younger groups as junior volunteers. Once they reach the age of eighteen, they become adult volunteers. This model provides a constant supply of help from individuals   who have benefitted already from attending such groups.

The   building is large and inviting.   It is decorated with bold colours and has comfy seating. It is a real home from home; a haven for families who have been disadvantaged by the closure of the life force of its community.

Martin and Jackie have clear ideas about how they wish to develop the Exodus Project but the lottery funding which they benefitted from is no longer available. Sadly, they have had to close two of their clubs due to lack of funding. This decision wasn't taken lightly. They do have two charity shops which raises some money and they obtain some funding from outside organisations for the use of their facilities. However, this is clearly not enough to keep their clubs, weekend activities and building going to cater for the ever growing number of children who are benefitting from the work being undertaken here.   Neither does it allow for future development.

Exodus do have a Just Giving page which can be found here if you wish to help further their work https://www.justgiving.com/exodus

In addition, you can keep up with activities on their Facebook page here

https://www.facebook.com/search/top/?q=the%20exodus%20project%20barnsley&epa=SEARCH_BOX

If anyone wishes undertake an event like The Three Peaks - or run a marathon to raise funds for Exodus - then Martin or Jackie would be pleased to hear from you. This will enable their vital work in the community to continue.

Contact them through their website to be found on www.exodusproject.org.uk.

Other books by this author include:

Osteoarthritis and Pain

The MND Diet: using nutrition to slow down the progression of the disease

The Alzheimer's and Vascular Dementia Disease Diet

The Asthma Diet

The Lymphoedema Diet

The EDS and Hypermobility Syndrome Diet

The EDS Recipe Book

The Osteoporosis Diet

Gastroparesis

Treatment Strategy for Migraine

The Reluctant Bowel

Angioedema

The Psoriasis Diet

The Anti Virus Diet (includes sections on coronavirus)

The Metabolic Syndrome Diet

And many more health related topics sold world-wide on Amazon

For more health tips follow Lynne on her blog

Quintessentially Lynne

And on Twitter @LynneDMNoble1